After a brief flirtation with zoology, in 1982, Tim became a doctor, first as a GP with an interest in many things, including complementary therapies and psychiatry. Listening to patients, their stories and their spirituality led him to become fascinated by palliative care. In 2002, Tim became a full-time palliative medicine physician. He has been a mountaineer for 50 years. He both loves and paints wild places.

For the numberless people I have tried to help and who have healed me in return.

Tim Harlow

THAT SOMETHING ELSE

A Reflection on Medicine
and Humanity

AUSTIN MACAULEY PUBLISHERS™

LONDON • CAMBRIDGE • NEW YORK • SHARJAH

A CIP catalogue record for this title is available from the British Library.

ISBN 9781398414679 (Paperback)
ISBN 9781398407640 (ePub e-book)

www.austinmacauley.com

First Published (2021)
Austin Macauley Publishers Ltd
25 Canada Square
Canary Wharf
London
E14 5LQ

There are many people who have contributed to this exploration and all have been important to me. The following have been especially pivotal: Becky Baines, Dickon Bevington, Patrick Cadigan, Jude Currivan, Paul Dieppe, Michael Dixon, Jim Gilbert, Johanna Harris, Sean O'Laoire, Therese Seward, Kieran Sweeney, Jim Swire, David Walford and Gill White. Your contributions have been priceless. The final work is, of course, my responsibility alone.

A Reflection on Medicine and Humanity

A doctor's personal exploration of spirituality and some other things, especially in relation to medicine, that from time to time bumps into religion in passing.

'Instead of insight, maybe all a man gets is strength to wander for a while. Maybe the only gift is a chance to inquire, to know nothing for certain. An inheritance of wonder and nothing more.'

– William Least-Heat Moon, *Blue Highways*

Table of Contents

Introduction

A thousand faces look up at the pulpit of the cathedral. Standing there is a doctor: no priest this and he not a religious man but instead deeply uncertain of many things. Yet this winter evening he is charged with sharing some reflections of his work as a doctor with this congregation. This is a hospice memorial service dedicated to many that have lost, or are losing, people they love. This special service is to help people remember, to grieve and to share that grief and loss with others. This doctor has no qualification to offer anyone religious help or even much certainty: there are others much better placed to offer that. All he can do is to share his understanding of the connections that we have as human beings. He has also noticed fleeting glimpses of particular moments or insights chanced upon and that seemed precious to him at the time.

Yet, surprisingly, this attempt to compress a professional lifetime of observing people confronted by illness and death into just ten minutes seems to strike a chord with many people. They come up to me at the end in tears, talk or write afterwards and say how good it is to hear a non-religious voice talking about such things. Even more unexpected are the priests and others with clear religious faith who say how important it is to find a spiritual language that can reach some of those who cannot deal with organised religion.

This original talk briefly tried to explore the usual understanding of hospice work; of a team of people, each with special skills working to control symptoms of those with life limiting illness in the community, hospice, and hospital. This aspect is all true and important with tremendous strength. But the main focus was on 'That Something Else' which was found in these places when people were attempting to help other people facing death and dying. It was this attempt to explore the ill-defined, powerful, and deep underpinnings of the ordinary business of medicine and healthcare that seemed to resonate so much. Some people wanted to hear more about this area which is not often talked about in medicine. Hence this book and its title.

Those looking for certainty, for revelation of truth and for clarity had best stop reading now. I am no guru or sage. Nor is this a quiet distillation of a completed journey with easy answers and I hope there is rarely any judgement. This is an exploration not an autobiography and so does not lend itself to a clear chronological order. My primary teachers have been the numberless people with illnesses, trauma and grief that I have met and been privileged to sit with and to stare together into the darkness for a while.

There are many scholarly works that review the literature and I will not replicate those although I have acknowledged quotes where possible. There are uncounted meetings, insights and chance conversations which, while sometimes only half remembered, have all contributed. Some words have cropped up often or been especially prominent and occasionally I have used these as chapter titles. There is much overlap of course between headings but I have used them more as lenses to illuminate a particular area than as clear demarcations. I have wandered across time and place and felt free to use whichever metaphor or method seems to illuminate the journey best at the time.

This is an honest attempt to portray one doctor's journey in medicine so far.

Chapter 1

Sacred Ground

'How could we have missed it? How could we have passed it by? There, right under our noses, all the time! Sacred space? It is us. It is the Self.'

— Stephen Wright and Jean Sayre-Adams

'This,' he said, 'this is sacred ground.'

David gestured round at the hospice ward in all its ordinariness. Nurses answered bells, volunteers brought cups of tea to a family at a bedside, a doctor on the phone gave advice about drug dosage to a colleague in a patient's home 20 miles away and a cleaner mopped something up from the floor. A new patient was wheeled into the ward by an ambulance crew who were taking extreme care to be as gentle with her as possible while appearing not to try at all. David saw the question in my face.

'It's not the place itself, it's what happens here, what people do and how they do it. Maybe we see it as God's work, maybe not. Still sacred ground.'

For a chaplain, quite a high church one at that, to say such a thing, to use those words, was powerful.

He set me thinking. I do not have the concept that he had of an all-powerful and all-knowing God whose work we might be doing. If I had considered the idea of sacred ground at all, then I would have thought of churches or cathedrals, maybe mosques and temples too. Maybe I would have thought about some ancient holy sites, hallowed by millennia of devotion. But not a ward in hospital or hospice.

Shortly after that conversation I was asked to see a couple in the General hospital next door to the hospice. They were trying to decide whether to continue with a treatment that had once been very helpful but by now was doing very little good. There was a real chance that further treatment would merely prolong his dying rather than enhance his life. They wanted to talk the whole thing through with a palliative care doctor. I was directed by the ward sister to a small curtained off alcove: it was in the corner of the usual supremely functional NHS general ward with attendant noise, bustle, smells and beeping machines. In truth I was a little irritated by the request which had come after I had already returned from the hospital and had other things on my mind but I knew that I could look professional enough and do the job adequately.

Behind the curtain was another world. It can be a cliché to call people beautiful, and for sure no one looks their best lying ill in a hospital bed or sitting up all night beside it. But this couple had created something very beautiful in that desperately ordinary place. Their love and respect for each other was immediately palpable. They openly acknowledged that he had only a short time to live and wanted to neither artificially prolong nor shorten his life. She was helping him to explore what options they had with a light and gentle touch that was as serious as death but never solemn.

My irritation dissolved instantly. For 45 minutes I was privileged, and that is the right word, to be allowed into this loving, heartfelt discussion. They cried, laughed and listened to one another, and to me, with a gracious attention and calm. There was a great sadness in the place, with great love and joy too. Their faith did not fit into any of the usual defined categories, but there was a deep sense of connectedness with something greater than any of us individually, but they did not need to name it.

It seemed a transition like night and day to re-enter the world of the hospital ward that had been only a curtain away from the place they had created. Walking away from the ward after this remarkable encounter, it was clear that I had been allowed a glimpse of something very important. These were ordinary people who, in extraordinary circumstances, had managed to make that mundane space, that ground, special, to make it sacred. Despite the gravity of what was being discussed and the imminence of death, I was left with the suspicion that if indeed there is a heaven, it may have something of that place about it. I realised that David was right: in a very real sense I had been on sacred ground. Another aspect to this experience that struck me was how I, in all my ordinariness, had been a part of this and even been able to contribute something worthwhile to this sacred ground.

More recently I was discussing with another priest, a hospice chaplain as well, the value of the brief conversation a patient and I had just had. The patient was a Christian and my part in the discussion had mainly been to witness and affirm her belief. Despite my agnosticism this seemed to me an important and valid way of walking with the patient on their journey for a while. The patient felt the way we discussed her religion amounted to a Christian gathering of a sort, with God in there. I suggested that it could be viewed as sacred ground, the place where such a thing could happen. The chaplain smiled and said, 'Yeah, it all counts.'

So what then is sacred ground? Is it a meaningful concept for doctors?

Sacred ground and Holy Ground are terms used sometimes interchangeably, and I would have used them so until made to think about it. Religions have clear ideas of Holy Ground: formally created as in consecrated ground as found in a church or temple, or made so by important religious events or meaning associated with a place. A glance around the British countryside shows that ideas of sacred places, of holy ground, are all around us. From the first humans following the retreating ice sheets north making barrows and henges right up to our current churches, mosques or temples. Churches and temples are often based in ordinary houses as well as in purpose-built buildings of all sizes and degrees of grandeur. There are legal definitions in England, both in the law of the land and canonical law, about sacred ground. These laws state how such status is conferred and deal with what can and cannot be done on such land, and by whom. These laws are highly relevant if, for instance, someone wishes to scatter the ashes of someone close to them or to bury a body on sacred ground. Matters such as exhumation of human remains are also strictly regulated. This is all important under certain circumstances but outside the scope of this discussion.

An obvious reason for religious people to call somewhere Holy Ground is because God has said it is so. Both the Bible and the Quran record instances of God telling people to remove their shoes for they are walking on Holy Ground. So for the religious such places need no more justification: they are Holy because God says they are Holy. Other places have become Holy because of extraordinary things believed to have happened there – miracles, visions, death or burial of important religious figures. Often humans built on these important places to reflect these events. Long association and veneration can amplify this enormously, as in the Western Wall in Jerusalem, The Golden Temple at Amritsar or the Kaaba at Mecca. Some churches in the UK are sited on previously sacred places from pre-Christian times, and other such sites can be made holy by ritual, blessing or consecration in some way.

So choosing to walk with another and using their metaphor, as discussed in the chapter on prayer, is easy enough. Much the same principles apply to Holy Ground and any doctor could choose to work with the patient's concept of what is Holy if that was helpful to the patient. But the boundary between Holy Ground and sacred ground seems at times blurred to me. When I was asked to talk in a conventionally holy place – Exeter cathedral – about working in a hospice and the idea of people making somewhere very ordinary into somewhere sacred made me focus on this grey area.

Linked with the concept of Sacred Ground is the idea of ritual. Different people in different contexts have noted how widespread ritual is over recorded history (and probably prehistory too, although we cannot ever know) and throughout the world, appearing as it does in all cultures. There seem to be very powerful reasons that ritual has always been so prevalent. At a certain level it can be explained as the spurious linking of certain actions with a particular result. Perhaps a hunting group checked their equipment in a certain way before setting off – a very practical act – but also asked for help from a particular spirit or god and after a few successful hunts relied on the same rituals to help them again.

Whether it is true that our brains are hard wired to seek out or use rituals is a moot point but it is undeniable that we do use them very widely, even in a secular society. We receive university degrees at ceremonies, we bury bodies according to certain customs, welcome people into our homes or societies in particular ways. Marrying one another contains certain rituals, and the military the world over make great use of rituals to foster comradeship and common values. Watch a professional rugby player about to take a penalty or conversion and very often they clearly use a set ritual that they have come to associate with success in that most public of situations.

Even in normal medical practice, ritual has a part to play. Much of the physical examination performed by doctors is, at least in part, to do with arcane ritual performed for reasons beside the chance of actually finding important physical signs. Even the verb we often use to describe the process, 'performing' an examination has an echo of ritual, of theatre. Certainly physical examination started out as a way of systematically searching for important information, and still has that important function, but the ritual has its own power as well both for patient and for doctor.

"The doctor didn't even examine me" is a frequent and deeply felt complaint.

It is important, of course, for the very good and practical reason that vital information about a condition may thus be missed and the patient has an excellent right to be aggrieved. But it also is that the patient feels that the doctor has not valued the patient, not fulfilled their side of the bargain implicit in the relationship and not honoured the ritual. It counts for very little if a doctor points out that an examination in the particular condition suspected would be very unlikely to provide useful information and going straight to, say, a scan would be much better. Something visceral and fundamental has been violated by not performing the ritual.

Some of the same driving forces that that power ritual also come into play with sacred ground. For somewhere to be considered holy ground there has to be a shared consensus in a group of people that the ground is indeed holy for whatever shared reason or belief. So too with sacred ground even if the term is not always explicit. More than one person has to see or feel, however unconsciously, that what happens there has something very special about it which is out of the ordinary. I do not think that the couple I referred to early on in this chapter, who, it seemed to me, had made the curtained off alcove into sacred ground thought about it in those terms. But I do know that they recognised that something out of the ordinary and critically important was going on.

How much does this matter? Is this all merely a way of helping those doctors who happen to think in this way anyway to reflect on an important aspect of their work? Maybe. Even at that level there is something here of value to help us deal with the extremes of human experience that we find ourselves immersed in and working with.

But there is something here of value to all of us healthcare workers, secular or religious or uncertain, if we start to be aware of it. If you accept, and it seems to me that there is good reason to do so, that there are levels of communication between human beings which are especially valuable in healthcare and which can be very helpful, but which do not sit easily in our normal model of medicine, then other things follow.

First is the idea that some places and some situations may facilitate such communication. In the same way that TS Eliot suggests in Little Gidding that some places retain a special significance to the Christian – 'You are here to kneel where prayer has been valid.'

So might some places become altered by the resonances of the interactions there repeated over time? Giving mind to that possibility, to even nurturing it and considering its enhancement, might be important in the collective culture of places where healthcare is given. Hospices are often aware of this importance at some level and encourage positive contributions to the place from various sources. Encouraging volunteers to work with flowers for instance, to make coffee for people or tend the garden works not just at the level of making pleasant surroundings, important though that is, but also helps contribute to this deeper resonance of the place.

Second is the recognition that these sacred spaces may be best viewed as temporary, produced by the moment and the people involved but nonetheless real and important for that. Would a cramped office on the edge of a hectic general ward be made sacred space permanently by doctors having an important, heartfelt, compassionate discussion with relatives or patient there? Maybe not. It might well be best to recognise the power of the human interaction to just last long enough to help at the time. But there is too the power of what Richard Selzer called "the cumulative murmuring".

So, just maybe over time, it can alter the feel of somewhere, to affect the deep resonance of a place.

Even if you accepted something of my suggestions above, it would be legitimate for you to question if the places where healthcare takes place are always sacred ground; must they always be considered as somewhere special or can they be neutral, or even malign? I am fortunate enough to have no experience of healthcare or healing interactions in truly dreadful circumstances – such as in a concentration camp. Exceptional people, such as Primo Levi, have managed to produce something good out of even such places but I am wholly unqualified to comment on whether there can be anything in such a situation that can be called sacred ground by any definition: the best I can do is to remain silent on this.

The less extreme situation of neutrality is another matter. A wholly routine intervention performed in a mechanical manner by someone "just doing their job", such as a vaccination, signing of a repeat prescription or checking blood pressure, might be of great value to someone and reduce the chances of bad things happening to them. Does that indifference of the act, even with a 'good' outcome, somehow affect any contribution to sacred ground?

Another less extreme situation, where a caring interaction is carried out by someone perhaps severely depressed or burnt out, perhaps even psychotic, might still have some echo of care for another, even if it is the care of the patient for the doctor. The idea of healing being a two-way process might extend to this too. Perhaps if there is complete mutual indifference, even mutual hostility, then the place where that occurs can be better considered a howling wilderness rather than sacred ground – whatever statistical lowering of risk or success of procedure results from the interaction.

One source of the difficulty of discussing sacred ground is asking what is the point of recognising this concept? Does it matter and is it in the end just an arcane discussion about something irrelevant?

It matters in two ways.

First, this can work at the level of just making us think about the healthcare environment, the culture – and it is clear that alone would be reason enough for it to matter. To attend carefully to the places where we work and heal one another is to attend to what happens there and the people who are on both sides of the interaction. At even this level of considering sacred space can be a proxy for valuing very important and often neglected aspects of care. So this would help us to look at the physical environment – beauty, architecture, colour, light, influence of nature – which is clearly too often shouldered aside by the supremely functional health care machines so much in vogue. Of course there has to be efficiency, ease of cleaning, flexibility of workspace and disinfection; and the reality of budget constraints with the need to get value for money is inescapable. But there need not be the either/or choice that we seem to accept now. And even modest improvement in staff morale might improve retention rates and reduce sickness. Might it improve health outcomes? Very likely and there is work done looking into this.

In their excellent book Sacred Space, Wright and Sayre-Adams identify the importance of such sacred space to rediscover a sense of meaning to facilitate recovery from burnout in medical practitioners. They do not consider the spiritual care of practitioners as some sort of optional extra; it is regarded as central to medical practice. They write movingly about a delegate to a conference on spirituality and health who said how difficult she found it to consider the spirituality of others in an organisation where she felt so neglected herself.

"It was a place where healing had been sacrificed on the altar of cost-effectiveness. 'How can I go back to work,' she asked, 'when my heart and soul are not welcome there?'"

If we accept that the heart and spirit of practitioners, and of patients, are important, then recognition of sacred space seems a helpful way to help create healthier place to care.

Second, there really do seem to be places where either so much good or so much harm has occurred that something has seeped into the fabric of the place. Many people find certain places have some sort of echo of the past about them. To recognise that hospitals, hospices and clinics have many episodes of great, often overwhelming human distress occurring in them is self-evident. Terrible news is broken, people die in bad circumstances and are treated for appalling injuries and illness in all such places. To recognise that and strive to still see, and seek the sacredness in them is very important.

So David was right, the hospice was sacred ground. The concept may not sit easily with some of our notions about healthcare, but we ignore that at our patients' peril, and at our own peril too.

Chapter 2
Healing

'Living matter, while not eluding the "laws of physics" as established up to date, is likely to involve other "laws of physics" hitherto unknown, which, however, once they have been revealed will form just as integral a part of this science as the former.'

– Erwin Schodinger,
What Is Life? The Physical Aspect of the Living Cell.

If, as a young doctor I ever considered the question, I would have assumed healing and curing to mean more or less the same thing. Of course we talked about a wound or a fracture healing rather than curing and an infection being cured not healed but otherwise there seemed no real difference. As doctors we were in the business of curing or healing people and that was that. Like any doctor I soon saw plenty of occasions when cure was impossible but still did not think about the etymology of these terms we used so freely.

Eventually I was forced to think much more carefully about this. Michael Dixon was, and still is, a GP in the same practice as me and a few years my senior. He is one of the most thoughtful people I have ever met. He also was very interested in complementary medicine. I had dabbled a little in hypnotherapy and was impressed by the results of some of the therapies I had seen my patients use, such as homeopathy and herbal medicine. I'd learnt to use the term Complementary Medicine as this suggested that both my conventional medicine and these other therapies were both trying to help people and should work together. This still seems to me a much more fruitful term than Alternative Medicine – implying that someone had to choose between two competing alternatives with no overlap. I had developed good working relationships with some local complementary practitioners and over time we had come to trust each other – to my patients' benefit.

As in other fields, some of the most vocal people have the least useful to say, with deeply entrenched positions on both sides. For example, I have met people who genuinely believed that all doctors had been somehow 'got at' during medical school so that even though we knew that there were effective ways to cure, say, cancer, we chose not to in order to keep up our collective professional front and keep in a job.

Often the drug companies were included in this conspiracy theory. They would be accused of constantly lying and suppressing inconvenient information to make money. Whilst some amoral multinational companies, such as some tobacco companies have indeed behaved like this, most pharmaceutical companies and the people who work in them are trying to do more good than harm as well as be profitable businesses.

It is true that doctors and researchers are fallible human beings and that we sometimes do become blinkered in our approach and indeed research fraud does exist. But to distort that into the revolting travesty described beggars belief. They were actually saying that as doctors we were prepared to let our friends and families suffer and die, knowing we could save them but choosing not to, just to prop up our charlatan profession and the profits of drug companies. Profoundly insulting.

There are also plenty of conventionally trained doctors who dismiss anything that does not fit into their understanding as quackery. Some complementary therapists do indeed greatly overplay their hand and make very extravagant claims. Yet it seems to me profoundly unscientific to reject all of them out of hand merely because they do not fit within our reductionist model.

Michael had been curious enough to attend a Spiritual Healing course and then invited the healer who had helped run the course, Gill White, to our practice journal club. Gill preferred the term Healer rather than Spiritual Healer but seemed less bothered about terminology and more about trying to open our minds to something she had seen to be very valuable. She talked in a very understated and gentle way, respectful of our model of healthcare and the work we did. Indeed, she had worked for some time with our local pain clinic and demonstrated how well these different models could work together to help people with chronic pain.

That hour or so of journal club changed me as a doctor and as a human being. I guess the time was right and the interactions I had seen and experienced with patients had started to chip away at my simplistic biomechanical views. It started to dawn on me: it was not necessary to choose either the standard medical model or healing, they could be combined. The most memorable moment for me was when I asked Gill if she was a bit apprehensive talking to a bunch of traditional doctors on their own turf.

'No,' she said, 'there are people who are holding me in white light at the moment and that helps.'

Blimey, I thought, there really is something very different going on here.

We ended up agreeing with Michael's proposal for a pragmatic study of healing in the surgery. Gill and a colleague would see patients the doctors had referred and who we felt we had done all we could to help. These were patients who had already been as fully investigated as was necessary to be sure we were not missing some serious treatable problem. We had done as much as we conventionally could. Some had either a chronic or relapsing condition, such as recurrent, very severe, cold sores or a wound that would not heal. Some did not fit into our normal neat diagnoses but were still clearly troubled.

57 patients were seen over the course of the study. Significant numbers of them improved where we had been unable to help them. Sometimes they were people who we had despaired of ever being able to help. Yet most of them found the healing welcome and helpful: many, but not all, of these apparently intractable problems improved significantly. It was surprisingly easy to suggest the idea of healing to patients and they generally did not seem to feel upset by the idea. In fact, the patients generally loved it.

One of the biggest surprises was how ordinary and how wholly unremarkable the whole process seemed. There were no flowing robes, no strange rites and no need to believe in any particular faith. Gill and her colleague Therese just got on with seeing people and seemed completely at ease in the surgery. If any of the doctors really did not want to understand any more about what the healers did, or if they thought it was all nonsense, the healers did not press the point but just got on with helping people as best they could.

But those of us who did want to understand more were very welcome to attend their sessions and to learn more about how healing can help. This was another step on my journey of understanding the place of spirituality in medicine. It was interesting to see that the patients in the healing trial also stopped coming to see their doctors as much in the year after the healing course. This was fascinating both for the practical benefits to the surgery – more doctor appointments available, and for the possibility that our medical model had its limitations.

Doctors come in all varieties and we are good, or less good, in different ways and at different times. Some are truly excellent while viewing humans as just complicated machines that need fixing and that are best understood when broken down into component parts. Others view things very differently. But all good doctors have one thing in common: they care. It matters to them when people suffer and it is more than just a purely intellectual exercise. I clearly see how that care, that rapt attention to the person and their story overlaps with the process of healing as understood by Gill and Therese – it is what all of us in healthcare do, consciously or unconsciously, if we are any good.

And this also means that we healthcare workers, including of course doctors, can actively cultivate this side of our interactions with people. This is emphatically not about giving even more of yourself. In fact, a crucial part of the recognition of healing is realising that we can help people and act best when we become channels for whatever is going on, not the source. When healing acts best, we specifically get out of its way and let it work where it should.

This then leads to the question, 'What is healing?' and thence to the next question, 'Where does it come from?'

I have no real idea.

There's the rub. Even starting to think about this area immediately pitches us into areas loaded with metaphor, false certainty, inadequate language, entrenched belief systems and very high emotion. This word "Healing" is inexact and few people seem to agree what it means. How can I discuss healing with someone whose ideas of this are entirely bound up with their faith and world view if I do not share their position and view?

This was brought home to me starkly very early on when a local clergyman, a generally open and helpful person – began to warn the congregation about our healers, considering that all healing should take place in the church. He feared that it was in some way dangerous if it took place outside of the Church. Later when I tried to introduce healing into our local hospice there were similar concerns and fears: real worries about false hope, undermining of belief and somehow sneaking in a particular faith or belief under the radar.

Yet how can I give confident reassurance that healing is not threatening without clear definitions, without the widespread acceptance of a working model? Looking at some of the claims made by some proponents of healing where there is talk of "energies… vibrations" really does not help much either. It can even get in the way as no one seems able to measure these things conventionally and this spurious exactitude simply will not stand up to scientific scrutiny.

Many complementary treatments come up against a similar problem. Proponents can be so keen to get acceptance by the healthcare system and become a recognised part of healthcare that they either make extravagant claims or almost sell out to the conventional paradigm and try to explain their therapy purely in scientific language. But maybe there is something going on which is not easily described or quantified but which I see as effective and real: yet attempting to capture it in our net of reductionist evidence may actually allow something very important to escape.

Sometimes too the unquestioning rejection of healing by scientists can be as much an emotional reaction as anything else. Science, for all its glorious power, is more subjective than we like to believe. When randomised controlled and blinded experiments are done with distant healing, as in the Targ and Byrd studies, the positive results were dismissed as impossible. Similarly, in Sheldrake's studies showing the reality of telepathy, the results are dismissed as impossible by some. A better answer might be that they are not impossible, merely incongruent with our normal thought paradigm, or as Ludvik Fleck suggested, our thought collective. More on that in due course.

I have come to understand four main ways that my acceptance of healing as a reality in my medical practice has been helpful. Inevitably there is overlap between these categories but they are a practical way to start talking about a complex subject.

First, healing provides an extra point of referral, a further treatment option. Doctors cannot easily choose who comes to see them, and with what problem. Even specialists will inevitably sometimes find a problem that presents in their area, perhaps a back pain or abdominal symptom, but then has ramifications and overlap with other areas. GPs (family doctors) of course see wholly unfiltered presentations of all sorts of problems and conditions, the vast majority of which the GPs deal with themselves. Some of these conditions do fit well into a biomedical model, such as treating a person's thyroid deficiency or arranging to have a hernia repaired, so are managed largely using that model.

Conventional scientific biomedical medicine is very good indeed at a lot of things, but not all. A crucial part of a doctor's job is identifying which of the many conditions they see – especially urgent, life threatening or life changing ones – are best handled this way. Our training is, rightly, very much geared to this recognition process and the subsequent management of such conditions. However, much of what doctors, especially family doctors, see presenting in their patients does not fit so neatly into this model. Once it is clear that either the condition the patient now has is not one that is best dealt with conventionally, or all reasonable conventional investigations and treatments have been been used, then the consultation between patient and doctor enters different territory, one of great uncertainty.

This place is very interesting and potentially very difficult for both parties. For convenience here I'll call it the 'Territory'. But before looking at that territory, we need to understand some of the normal, but often unacknowledged, assumptions that people make when playing the role of doctor or of patient.

The unspoken bargain made when a patient sees a doctor runs something like this. The patient agrees to be reasonably honest with the doctor, give them the information they need and they then expect to have their disease or condition understood and cured, or at least diagnosed and managed. The doctor in turn expects the patient to be honest and allow them access to sometimes very personal information, submit to examination and investigation to allow a diagnosis leading to a management plan with which the patient will co-operate. Clearly there are some situations, for example with the management of drug or alcohol addiction or a few psychiatric conditions, where the assumptions are necessarily different for both patient and doctor. However, most people, when they play the roles either of patient or doctor, implicitly acknowledge these assumptions and the resulting goodwill makes the consultation workable.

The 'Territory' can become very uncomfortable for everyone involved. It seems to each party, to patient and to doctor, that, the implicit bargain has been broken: people can feel betrayed and angry. A specific example might be a patient who feels tired, irritable and with low mood. The doctor might acknowledge the distress the patient feels but decides it is not a serious depressive illness or some other treatable underlying condition. They might well not offer medication, or maybe they will suggest exercise or sleep hygiene. They might even offer an antidepressant drug. In any event they feel they have done their honest best and thereby fulfilled their obligations in the unspoken bargain.

Perhaps the patient will be content with whatever the doctor has offered and all is well. But either at that consultation, or more commonly, after a series of consultations about the same problem, the patient feels the doctor has not kept their side of the bargain. They have told the doctor what is wrong, done what the doctor suggested and yet things stay the same, maybe with the addition of unwelcome side effects from ineffective medication. The doctor for their part begins to feel upset as the patient seems not to be fitting into the usual medical model of illness and "ought" to have got better by now; they may doubt if the symptoms described are actually "real".

Sometimes this gets to the stage of the doctor dreading seeing the patient again because the whole process seems so unfruitful – one reason for the so called 'heart-sink patient' where the doctor's heart sinks when they see the patient's name on the list for that surgery. In reality it is not generally the patient themselves who causes a sinking heart, it is the disconnect between what the doctor perceives they can offer and the difficulty and intractability of the symptoms the patient experiences.

There are ways out of this impasse. Sometimes the patient resolves things by voting with their feet and seeing another doctor or other therapist. They may just accept the limitations of what the doctor can offer. The doctor may also draw a clear boundary and make it clear to the patient what they can offer and what they cannot offer. These approaches generally work well enough and are used a great deal although sometimes at the cost of mutual dissatisfaction.

But I described this 'Territory' as interesting. If the doctor recognises the consultations have reached this territory then the extra point of referral available from healing and some other therapies comes in. This is not just fobbing off the patient by sending them somewhere else, but rather it is a recognition of both the reality of the patient's suffering and the limitations of the conventional medical model. Due to the inherent imbalance of power in the doctor patient relationship it generally requires the doctor to initiate this process.

This can never be a one-way process – people are human and make mistakes. Things change, illnesses evolve and there is a crucial advantage in the doctor remaining involved in this process and being able to restart or intensify medical management if it should be necessary. So a doctor may agree with a patient that the current condition may best be helped by using healing to augment the body's natural healing mechanisms. However, they are wise also not make the patient feel abandoned and arrange some kind of follow up, even by email or phone, to maintain involvement.

This reframing and understanding of the natural history of a consultation can be transforming. Instead of dreading that moment when the doctor realises that they cannot help this person with conventional medical means (or the patient glumly works that out for themselves), it can become a real chance to offer positive help where none existed before and for relationship to be maintained.

The second way in which I found my acceptance of healing to be so helpful is more matter of fact. There is a significant appetite for CAM (Complementary and Alternative Medicine) in the UK and many people use various therapies either alone or in combination with conventional ones. They and their friends often will have found the CAM practitioners helpful, interested, and may indeed have developed long term relationships with them.

But they don't tell their doctors. There is evidence that they do not like to offend us as doctors and they can also feel embarrassed. If we as doctors make it clear that we respect their choices, want to work with others and are not engaged in some sort of futile turf war with other therapies they are more likely to tell us what else they are doing. They will also be more likely to receive our ideas positively and if we have, with their permission, discussed their case with a CAM practitioner who they trust – even better.

This paradoxical effect is important. If I as a doctor am clear about how I can help, but open to patients' ideas and respectful of those who they have found useful to them, then the patient is more likely not just to tell me about their thoughts but to listen to my advice too. A good example is of a family who accepted my advice about vaccination after initially being reluctant because of the advice of a local homeopath. After my discussing it with the homeopath we agreed to disagree but the fact of my understanding and respecting their position was far more persuasive that my merely dismissing it all as unscientific.

The third way healing has helped me is less obvious and more subtle. In conventional treatment we are taught about diseases, injuries and their treatments – many of which treatments are very powerful and effective. This has been and will always remain my starting point in my medical work, and I believe it would be a very unwise doctor who started anywhere else: what is wrong and what should I do about it?

Many CAM practitioners view things differently. They look at the illness very much in the context of the person with the condition. This thinking very much about the person (not just obvious things such as their renal function or allergies for instance) and what treatment is right for them is very useful for us conventionally trained doctors to remember. So attempting to individualise treatment is worthwhile. How can we do that beyond acting out a meaningless platitude?

It started for me by getting a feel for which of my conventional colleagues I should refer a patient of mine to with a particular problem. This was relatively easy with conventional colleagues I had got to know. This patient would like a no-nonsense approach – this one needed a gentler pair of hands even for a relatively straightforward matter such as a hernia repair or a new hip.

But I also developed a feel for which sort of complementary approach or practitioner would be good for a particular person to see. This took time to develop but was in the end really helpful. I found that I was developing a feel for what therapy or therapist suited a particular person. This process developed over years and was also a helpful side effect for myself when choosing conventional treatments to use for various conditions. Of course there are good evidence-based guidelines for lots of treatments but even guidelines have some flexibility. How long to persist with exercise and weight loss when considering high blood pressure treatment before using medication is an example.

The last way I noted acceptance of healing as reality had changed my practice was the most fundamental. It changed me.

I have not mentioned the term spirituality so far in the context of healing. Although this approach does allow healing specifically to be discussed as related to medical matters, it is incomplete: spirituality is there in any consideration of healing. If, as I suggest, spirituality involves the search for meaning, perhaps with transcendence and wholeness, or connectedness, then much of healing will involve spirituality and vice versa. One clear demonstration of this is to look at healing in palliative care. At first glance the idea of 'dying healed' seems a nonsense, an oxymoron and thus irrelevant to palliative care.

What is nonsense, and dangerous nonsense at that, is the idea of miracle cures, of healers being able to do wonderful things if only the doctors would stop all their dreadful poisons that they know are at best useless. People do indeed sometimes fare much better, and sometimes much worse, with a particular condition than we expect or can explain. All doctors at some time in their careers have seen a horrible disease fading away or stopping in its tracks for no reason we can understand. These are fascinating cases, and maybe under-investigated, but I am very wary of healing being invoked to claim a miracle cure.

With its name derived from the Latin 'pallium' (a cloak), palliative care is all about those conditions that we cannot cure, where all we can do is to treat symptoms and to cloak them. So healing used as a synonym for curing clearly no longer works. When people are faced with the incurable in themselves or those close to them, with the imminent dissolution of so much shared history and experience, then other aspects of healing really matter.

As well as 'making healthy' and 'overcoming disease', healing is also about bringing to an end or a conclusion – reconciliation. Healing involves integration and balance, honouring all parts of ourselves, our path through life and our relationships. These aspects of healing are absolutely central to holistic palliative care. So the idea of 'Dying Healed' is not such an odd thing as it first seems. Good palliative care, whether given by specialists, healthcare professionals in other fields or family and friends, must involve this healing. It might involve someone who explicitly acts as a healer, or more commonly by those playing their natural roles with rapt attention and care. So helpful here is that very particular kind of love which is properly found in medicine, and which merits its own chapter to discuss.

An extraordinarily clear description of one way in which this process of healing can happen is given by Tolstoy in *The Death of Ivan Ilyich.* Fiction, at any rate good fiction, is based on fact and truth. Nowhere have I seen truth expressed in fiction more clearly than in this little masterpiece of Tolstoy's. The disintegration of Ilyich's world, and world view, as his illness progresses is clear and very poignant. It mirrors a process that we see many people going through as they face terminal illness.

But Tolstoy, the Master of recording the human condition, also beautifully records the healing that Ilyich experiences at the end of his life.

'And all at once it became clear to him that what had tortured him and would not leave him was suddenly dropping away all at once on both sides and on ten sides and on all sides... he looked for his old accustomed fear of death, and did not find it. "Where is it? What death?" There was no terror, because death was not either.'

People may find nature, music, beauty, laughter, children, literature, colour, architecture and much else healing too and we must remember that when caring for them. And as I suggest when considering prayer, it is important to remember how healing is a two-way process. When we fully focus on another human being with the intent to help them, we are healed too. The boundary between what is prayer and what is healing seems to me very ill defined, and best kept that way.

Chapter 3

Prayer

'Prayer must never be answered: if it is, is ceases to be prayer and becomes correspondence.'

– Oscar Wilde

'How can you pray with him? You're no Christian even if he is. You don't even believe in God!'

This is not just a fair point about me, encapsulating as it does so much that I have worried about. It also strikes deeply into the entire question of spirituality, God and religion. At first glance it seems that any acceptance of meaningful prayer demands an acceptance of a divine being – otherwise who is it that is being prayed to?

Christianity, Islam and other mainstream religions look at prayer as a divinely ordered duty often with clear instructions about how and when it is to be performed. Interpretations vary but ideas about glorifying God, worship, supplication and intercession are very much part of the fabric of religions, with perhaps the exception of certain Buddhist traditions. Prayer is not viewed as an optional extra but as a fundamental duty.

Once I did fit into a such clear religious framework. Then, as a Christian who had accepted Jesus as my saviour, I believed in prayer as direct conversation with God. So prayer was entirely natural with endless guidance about how to do it from Christian sources. Even then prayer for me was not some sort of celestial shopping exercise; I understood that much. Even so, I believed in the "Power of Prayer" and in a God listening directly to me as an individual even if He did not, or could not, always answer prayers literally.

This view of prayer, with a faithful Christian believing in a meaningful interaction with a supreme being who at least cares deeply about both me and the conversation, is clear enough. There is obviously a very wide variation in acceptance of spiritual matters in different faiths, beliefs and world views. Even within a particular sect of a particular religion there is sometimes great diversity of views on important questions. Nonetheless, many people would be astonished that prayer was even considered by one who did not believe in God. No God means no prayer: easy.

A stark illustration of this came in my early 20s. Going round a cathedral I signed a petition of protest against the then Soviet Union's persecution of Christians. The volunteer attending the petition was incredulous that not only was I not a church goer, but an atheist.

'Do you know what you have just signed?'

'Yes, no one should be persecuted for their religion.'

'Well, I shall pray for you.'

This last almost in sorrow, and bemusement when I thanked her. A binary view indeed: either you are for a religion or you are against it.

I had indeed lost all faith completely. The detail of this journey is unremarkable and probably reflected in the story of many young people of that time. It is enough to say that by the time I was at medical school I was comfortable in my atheism. After some years of what Gandhi called 'traversing the desert of atheism', I emerged pretty clear that I was not a Christian, or indeed a follower of any other organised religion, and I was distrustful of anyone claiming to have clear religious answers.

During this time, the 1980s, the climate around religion in healthcare, and attitudes to it hardened. There was increasing suspicion of doctors or nurses expressing their own religion, and overt hostility to any attempt by professionals to impose their own beliefs on patients. Given the imbalance of power inherent in any health professional's relationship with someone ill or vulnerable that made complete sense to me. Nurses at this time understandably feared that they might lose their jobs for praying with patients.

Proselytising, with the risk of undermining someone's own beliefs, is completely wrong. There is no place for deathbed conversions despite the anxious desire of some strongly religious to do just that and "to save them". That seemed to me, and also to many others then, as no less than an assault. It seems that way to me still. The idea that someone who is dying is doomed to rot in Hell, unless they espouse one particular person's understanding of one particular brand of one particular faith before they die, is utterly revolting.

But it only fair to acknowledge that Religion has always been an important force steering people to choose to work in healthcare. Looking after the sick is specifically mentioned as God's will in many religions. Compassion for the sick is seen as very much God's work. I have come across many healthcare workers whose different religions are potent drivers for their excellent work. The Christian Medical Fellowship, for example, has over 4000 members.

But there are also lots of excellent and deeply compassionate doctors who are atheist or agnostic. They do not need a holy book to tell them what is right. I too was comfortable in my certainty that there was no God and the only purpose in life was what we as humans made for ourselves. Looking into the eyes of a suffering fellow human being was enough to give me that purpose.

Things changed. Experiences with life generally and with individual patients made me more aware of some of the complexity of the world. I saw there might well be times when spiritual needs might be helped or at least acknowledged and honoured by prayer. But as an atheist turned agnostic, I did not see how to do that without being disingenuous or risking the sack.

Medicine is full of difficult ethical and moral questions. Philosophers often use theoretical thought experiments to really drill down into important ethical questions. It is salutary that Julian Baggini, who is both an excellent philosopher and entertaining when communicating serious ideas, says that in everyday medicine there are so many important ethical questions that there is no need for theoretical models – real life questions are difficult enough.

It turns out that an excellent starting point when considering an ethical medical problem is to ask, 'Who gains out of this?'

This is not always as straightforward as I have stated it – what is a gain, how do you measure it, what timescale, is causality as clear as it seems – these are just a few points to consider. If a doctor does anything with or to a patient where their primary aim is not doing the patient more good than harm, then something is wrong. Having the primary aim as trying to help the patient does not guarantee doing the right thing but it is a good starting point. That same principle also helps me when considering prayer.

If a doctor prays with a patient at the doctor's instigation, to impose the doctor's beliefs on the patient, even if they believe they are saving the patient from great spiritual harm thereby, it is answering the doctor's agenda. That is to say that the patient is not the one who gains. Indeed, they may suffer considerable harm by having their own moral and spiritual framework questioned when they are extremely vulnerable and have no time or ability to rebuild another one.

But a patient asking for a doctor to pray with them and to give them spiritual solace may be wholly different – at least ethically. However helpful that is theoretically, it does not help much with the doctor who might feel very uncomfortable with such a request. Around the time of my medical qualification, I certainly was just such a doctor who would be deeply uneasy at the idea of prayer with a patient.

Sean O'Laiore was very helpful to me when I was thinking about this. Sean lives and ministers in California and describes himself as 'a heterodox Irish priest'. Whilst still a devout Roman Catholic priest, he sees his faith as a place to reach out from and not a place to defend. This openness to other views whilst still being clear about your own is something I have found very appealing in people from many different religious positions. Sean's advice was based on religions being "metaphors for that which is ineffable" and he was clear that choosing to use someone else's metaphor, to walk with them for a while, was, if your intent was good, a compassionate and correct thing to do. This was astonishingly liberating for me. If I prayed with someone it did not imply accepting, or even having an opinion about, their own religion but it was respectfully honouring both them and their understanding of the deeper questions of the human condition.

So now, over 40 years since starting medicine, prayer has become an accepted and normal part of my professional and personal life. But I am as far from personal acceptance of a specific religion as ever. I now see three broad and overlapping strands about using prayer in healthcare, and perhaps in other contexts too.

First, and maybe easiest to consider, is when someone has a firm belief in a particular religion and sees prayer as talking directly to God. They may consider that prayer and demonstration of faith can even influence God's actions in the world. This is a traditional view of prayer. Some people would find it hard to think of prayer in any other way. Even a doctor like me who cannot think of a micro-managing deity who can be appeased or influenced can still join in with that sort of prayer when it is appropriate, helps the patient, and it is at the patient's request.

This was the area I used to find hardest – if I could not really believe that there was a God as the patient understood it, was I somehow being untrue to myself and the patient if I went along with it? However, the idea that I could join with them, respect them and demonstrate that I wanted to walk with them for a while is, I believe, a good reason to put my own beliefs to one side for a while. It's not about me, it's about the patient. There is a power in ritual, in shared participation that may be immensely useful. Christians believe what Jesus was reported to have promised his disciples: 'For where two or three gather in my name, there am I with them.' So for me to choose to be with a patient, to make that gathering a reality for them, and so to help them feel the presence of their God seems an honour to me and not a problem.

Richard Dawkins is a towering zoologist whose ground-breaking book *The Selfish Gene* was very influential when I briefly flirted with zoology before medicine. It has proved to be still essentially correct and remains very important for me. Dawkins is an outspoken atheist but also describes himself as a 'cultural Christian' enjoying Christmas carols and services which he sees as part of his heritage. This shared culture, shared metaphor and ritual can still be a force for good.

Honesty is always important. When a patient asks me if I believe God can answer prayers and so cure people, then I will say that it does not matter what I think and my beliefs. What matters is them and their understanding which I just want to help with. If pushed it is also honest to say that I do not believe that is how prayer works and they are asking for a miracle, but maybe they know more than me about this. It is a fact that there are people with dreadful illnesses who do either much better, and sometimes much worse, than we as doctors expect – for no reason anyone can yet explain. So it is also honest to say that we always know less than we think we do. And it is also honest to say that I have heard people asking not for a cure, but for the strength to bear whatever God's will for them is; and that seems a good thing to pray to God for.

One worry I have is the risk of a patient persistently asking me my views on, for instance prayer. Usually this can be dealt with as above, or by deflecting with a statement such as, 'I am really interested in why you are asking me about this, why my views are so important when this is about you, not about me.'

Yet occasionally there will be someone who continues to push and where, in the end, only the bald truth will do. Then I guess the more doggedly a patient continues to push a question, the less likely they are to be harmed in some way by a gentle but clear disagreement with their view.

Hope is a fascinating and slightly slippery concept well worth discussing in its own right. In the context of prayer though it is enough to consider when the unvarnished brutal full truth may actually be an assault. Honesty; respectfully and compassionately honouring a person and their views, demands a nuanced and gentle recognition of where a person is in their understanding and their journey.

As in the breaking of bad news to a patient, considering how much of the truth to tell at a particular moment is right. Here it is of course still true that the test of "who gains from this" still applies. If I do not tell someone information because the process will be uncomfortable for me, that is a bad reason. If I am trying, however imperfectly, to give the whole truth, but in a manageable way that does not overwhelm the patient, that is different and honest. And the same principle will apply to a patient's enquiries about a doctor's beliefs.

There is a second way prayer is important. This has echoes of healing and of intention: what one person calls prayer another may call healing. Here I think there are levels of connection and of communication between human beings that are important and yet poorly understood. As discussed in the chapter on healing, I believe there is a power in the rapt and focussed attention of one person on another, and in its reciprocation. Prayer can certainly work at this level too and

47

the language and the metaphors we use in prayer and spirituality may allow access to levels of connection that I believe have an important part to play in medicine.

There is plenty of evidence that interventions by doctors (and other healthcare professionals) have powerful effects which are not explained by the standard pharmacology, anatomy and physiology that we normally rely on in medicine. These effects can be beneficial – placebo or harmful – nocebo. Both effects are increasingly understood to be very important in all medicine. It is established beyond doubt that, for instance, inert pills with no pharmacological action at all can have significant effects on both physical and mental illnesses. This is a vast and important area in its own right deserving of a great deal of attention. Paul Dieppe suggests that nocebo's harmful effects can be even more significant than the positive effects of placebo, taking some time and effort to undo the damage caused. In brief: it matters in prayer too.

This means that as well as working at a level of healing, which I believe to be a fact but some people dismiss as utter nonsense, there is a known, accepted and powerful way in which prayer may be really useful. We know that the body has its own healing mechanisms that work all the time dealing with infections, trauma, and probably even early cancers. If these systems are badly damaged, for instance by chemotherapy or some illnesses, then we may not be able to deal with even simple infections despite very powerful antibiotics.

We know that emotional trauma, such as bereavement, can markedly increase the rate of physical illnesses such as infections or heart disease. So anything that can help our bodies' natural healing mechanisms is worthwhile. Prayer can work at this placebo level as well and should be relatively uncontroversial in this context.

One of the things I have continually bumped into in my work, and which I finally now misunderstand a little less, is how the whole of medicine is not a one-way street. It is not the case that one group of people (doctors) does something – healthcare – to another group of people (patients). It is actually a two-way process. The truth is that we are just human beings helping, and being helped, at the same time. Early on in my medical training a particularly good doctor who is still a close friend told me:

'It is a sick doctor that is not healed by his patients.'

When we are in these remarkable relationships with patients, of which prayer may sometimes be a part, it can be good for us too.

So any idea that prayer is some sort of gift we can paternalistically give out is wrong. If we engage in prayer, for the good reasons outlined here and for the benefit of our patients, then maybe we will benefit too. Doctors do have a high rate of burnout, mental illness, suicide and alcoholism. If the health and well-being of doctors and other healthcare workers is also helped by these connections, by prayer, then that is good side effect.

A third way where prayer may be helpful is, for me, harder to pin down than the first two. I have already rejected the concrete certainties of religion (or of confident atheism for that matter) and think that the most likely outcome when I die is oblivion. But the universe is a complicated place and we understand only some of it. So it is possible that in the vast gaps in our knowledge there will be uncertainties and there may exist some thing or things that we do not comprehend.

In that place of unknowing there might be something that some people handle mentally by using a term – "God". Clearly to claim any one of our holy books, beliefs, religions or scriptures can accurately and completely portray this something in its entirety is, I suggest, hubris of the highest degree. However, we may find a working model that serves to help us on occasions. We might be able to connect with some aspect of a collective unconscious or some entity by using the metaphor of prayer. This word "God" is loaded with perhaps more baggage than any other in the English language but I use it in this context as a shorthand, a working model, for the complexities and uncertainties that I have been considering.

There are some specific examples where I have attempted this connection with the unknowable and where even an unreligious agnostic like me has found a place for prayer.

I have certified as dead hundreds of human bodies. It is one of the duties of a doctor that can be become routine and mechanical. Yes, there are specific and very important tests that must be done to ensure this is one diagnosis we never get wrong. But for me it never stopped being something that really mattered beyond the basic procedure. Sometimes the bodies were of strangers, living people that I had never known. But more often these were people that I knew, that I had seen breath, laugh, talk, cry, love. Sometimes they had been friends. They certainly once had all been someone's friend, lover, child, spouse, parent.

Once I had carried out my medical duty and determined for certain that this person had died the most natural thing for me was to say The Lord's Prayer to myself. If I knew they were of a specific faith or of no religion, I would instead say to myself something that might reflect or honour whatever I did know of them.

Often this would be, 'I'm grateful that in all the vastness of time and space our paths crossed and I wish you well with whatever journey you are now on.'

If there were relatives present during the certification process – a choice I always gave them after explaining what it would entail – they seemed content as far as I could tell, that I paused for a short time in respect. It was an extraordinary moment for them and it was right to let them know that it was to me more than just a dry medical matter.

I found doctoring very difficult at times – maybe most of us do. And on the way to a particularly awkward situation, such as a talking to a family who found it hard to believe that there really was no medical procedure that would do their relative more good than harm, I would ask for help.

Who from? No idea. And afterwards I tried to remember to say 'Thank you'. To whom? No idea.

I am certain there is no personal micromanaging God up in the sky answering me. I am revolted by the very idea of a God in the universe they created which is working to the rules they had made, and who had the power to help us in the dreadful situations inherent in that imposed order, but who chose not to help unless we asked really nicely. And maybe not even then. Neither does the idea of a parallel spirit world where benign ghosts of dead people can help us if we ask make any sense to me; although I know people who have exactly this view.

Just a frightened little human whistling in the dark? Maybe. Comforted by the shadow of a ritual learnt as a child? Maybe. Psychologically helped by the feeling that the Universe may not be wholly indifferent? Maybe all of these. And maybe beyond all that there might be a way that we can momentarily connect with something larger than ourselves, and part of ourselves; something perhaps Jung touched on when he referred to the idea of a "Collective Unconscious".

At one time I did not want to even consider using prayer as a doctor without clarity of what I was doing and why. Now I am content with my uncertainty, in this as in so much else. I'll use it, believe it to be worthwhile and do not need a rigid belief system to support it. The Buddha is reported to have compared the quest for such certainty in spiritual matters to a man wounded by an arrow who refuses any treatment unless he knows the name of the man who shot it, all the details of him and his family and the wood the arrow was made from. Similarly, I know so little, but can still recognise something worthwhile and use it.

Chapter 4

Love

'... Love is better than sacrifice.'
— Belden C Lane, *The Solace of Fierce Landscapes*

When I talk to people about love in medicine, especially when I suggest that the practice of medicine is founded on love, it can provoke interesting reactions. Surprise, suspicion, bafflement, and sometimes a smile and a nod. By many people's understanding of the word, the very idea of including love even as a tolerable component of good medicine seems at best naive, at worst disastrous. But the love I mean here, as the foundation of medicine, is of a very specific and carefully defined sort which is valuable in everyday practice.

It is worth setting the scene of this discussion by considering the concept of emotional granularity. This is where we use precise words to describe very specific and nuanced emotions, even borrowing words form other languages to do so when our own language fails us. This care in observing, labelling, and describing emotion can help us considerably to understand both our own internal world and also why we are reacting to something in a particular way. It may as well help us to communicate something of our internal world to others.

Emotional granularity seems even to have positive benefits for our mental health by enabling us better to understand why we are feeling a particular emotion which at first glance might seem very generalised. We may then gently enquire of our emotions to give insight into what may be more complex roots of our feelings, and in doing so allow us better to deal with them. Someone might simply say that they are feeling "low" and they may be troubled by that negative emotion without really being able to understand or address the causes of the emotion. If they can be helped to realise that they are feeling not just "low" but are in fact slightly frustrated, a little anxious and longing for something realistically unattainable then they may well be better able to deal with their negative emotion and their overall situation.

To give a concrete example: Saudade is a Portuguese word describing a melancholic longing or nostalgia for a person, place or thing that is far away in space or time. This may even be a vague dreaming wistfulness for phenomena that may not even exist. Such careful precision of meaning may help someone to understand their own feelings better and to give the emotion due recognition whilst understanding the roots of their feelings.

Thus it is also with love. The Ancient Greeks used at least six words for love and any discussion of love in a medical context could usefully start by considering these words even if none of them in the end actually fits the bill completely. The very act of defining categories of love must also acknowledge that there is considerable overlap between these types of love. For all my talk of emotional granularity, I do recognise that insisting on too rigid a separation of different sorts of love by definition will miss something important about the inherent fuzziness of both the human condition and the words we use to try and capture some of it. HG Wells observed this clearly when he noted that "the forceps of our minds are clumsy forceps and crush the truth a little in taking hold of it".

Eros is the type of love that many people fear love as used in medicine to mean. This sexual passion, romance and desire, celebrated on Valentine's day for instance, is often what people consider the word love to mean when used without qualification. It is also absolutely the kind of love most disastrous in medical matters. There is always an imbalance of power inherent in a doctor/patient encounter and recognition of this has led to rigorous exclusion of eros from medical matters. Whatever else love can usefully mean in a therapeutic relationship, it is not eros. Powerful ethical and legal barriers have been created to prevent eros entering into the medical relationship: this is a good thing and I do not propose weakening those barriers.

Philia refers to deep companionship or comradely friendship. This may happen in teams, and also in the military or on expeditions or other joint endeavours. Loyalty in shared adversity with reliance on each other can foster this feeling. It will rarely be significant in the therapeutic relationship but will certainly be relevant within medical or other healthcare teams. Medicine is rightly an increasingly collegiate matter and philia, provided it does not foster too much introspection and feelings of "them and us", can be both important and appropriate. But this is still not the foundation of medicine.

Ludus, a playful affection or frivolity is important in everyday life. Teasing, flirting, exuberance, gentle and well-intentioned banter, and laughter are part of the richness of life and to be celebrated. This does have a place in medicine but has to be used sparingly and with great care in any therapeutic context. Ludus is certainly not a foundation of medicine even if a carefully used playfulness may at times lighten a mood and allow the serious business of medicine to be a little less solemn.

Agape is an interesting candidate for love in medicine. It is that selfless love for humanity often referred to by different religions that each recognise this universal, unconditional kindness as important in the human condition. The different traditions may give it different names but the kindness to strangers it engenders is greatly enriching to human relationships. Agape is relevant to medicine and is a driver for much that is good in human relationships in general as well as in the specific case of medicine. The awareness of Agape, either the genuine feeling of it or the awareness of the duty to practice it, is sometimes a potent driver for people to choose to work in medicine in the first place. It may well be a powerful force keeping doctors working in sometimes very difficult circumstances. So I do think that Agape, that sort of unconditional love, is definitely a part of what I mean, a part of the foundation of medicine, but it is by no means all.

Pragma may be used a little differently now to how the Greeks used it but we today might consider it to be a slow burning, mature and growing love. This might be found in long established relationships. Literally, pragmatic, it involves the making of compromises with give and take to make things work. Although medicine does not always exhibit this kind of longer-term love, the relationship between a family doctor and their patients may well involve pragma.

Indeed, any doctor in a specialist field managing patients with chronic conditions over years or even generations, perhaps involving some neurodegenerative diseases, might find pragma an important component of their therapeutic relationship. The tacit acceptance of each other's humanity with all its faults and triumphs can be a beautiful thing. The doctor knows the patient as a four-dimensional person in the context of their surroundings and relationships and the patient knows the doctor as a fully drawn human being. Boundaries are still important but each person can find it easier to forgive the other their human frailties and to trust one another. There is more than pragma to the love that underpins medicine but it is an important component and certainly does have a place.

Philautia is at first glance an unlikely ingredient of medical practice. There is of course the narcissism, the self-aggrandising characteristic, which is the negative side of philautia. That is indeed a fault as common in medical people as in any other group of humans, perhaps at times more common despite the inevitable failures of even the cleverest medicine which can act as a guard against hubris. The arrogant side of philautia, which treats the therapeutic relationship as some sort of stage upon which the doctor performs for their own benefit, is likely to be unhelpful. Good medicine can sometimes still be done in that context, but great dangers await and there are plenty of cases where the whole supposedly therapeutic encounter becomes entirely about the doctor and the patient suffers – sometimes terribly. The rogue surgeon Ian Paterson's patients could warn us of the appalling dangers here.

But there is a quieter and more positive side of philautia which involves a healthy level of self-esteem with a comfort in one's own skin that enhances the ability to care for, love, and appreciate others. This is an important characteristic for doctors, and their long-term mental health, which is well worth cultivating. Given that burnout, psychiatric illness, addiction and early retirement are so prevalent amongst doctors, maybe something that specifically encourages doctors to value themselves as well as their patients should be encouraged. All doctors will see examples of their colleagues putting demands on themselves, in time, desire for perfection and meeting patients' needs, that they would never expect of others. So maybe philautia does have a place, a cautious but very real place, in medical practice. The health and well-being of doctors is worthwhile both because it is good for our patients and because it is right in itself. The NHS does not have a good record of caring for its own staff: this in an organisation whose very existence is fundamentally about caring for people. So encouraging doctors to care for and to value themselves is philautia well worth cultivating in a careful manner. It is not however the love that I mean as a foundation of medicine.

There are at least two further uses of the word love which can sometimes also cause confusion, although far less in this context and so worth a mention just for completeness.

"I love chocolate!" (Or wine or the colour pink or many other things that we crave and celebrate.)

This extreme form of liking is part of our normal parlance and harmless fun in context. A doctor may 'love' travelling to a particular hospital for a clinic for instance, where appropriate patients are carefully referred and the staff are pleasant and work in good, well-resourced surroundings where the doctor can do their job properly. All well and good, but this is not part the love I am considering.

The religious often talk of the love of God. This is clearly very important to consider in religious matters and theological discussions and even in the motivation of religious doctors. Religious love is by definition outside the realm of human love and beyond human understanding and so outside my discussion. It would clearly be important however for those considering their medical work to be a religious duty or expression of service to God. A religious doctor might well consider that if God still loves someone who is deeply flawed for instance, then they as a doctor have a duty to recognise that such a person is still important to God despite their shortcomings and so worthy of the doctor's best endeavours.

So having said what this elusive medical love I am talking about is not, and tried to define the limits of the involvement of various other recognised sorts of love, it is time to consider what love is in medicine.

A useful starting point to dig a little deeper into this question comes from the Christian theologian and medical ethicist Alastair Campbell. In his book *Moderated Love,* he begins to deal with the role of professions that have dealings with people in difficulties – medicine certainly fits the bill here – and the possible conflict between the need to earn money and yet offer an ideal of care. He argues that because these professions deal with people when they are especially vulnerable and unable to help themselves that there is a need for "… the addition of love to the quest for monetary gain".

Campbell's 'moderators of love' include a kind of supervisory role to even out power and so to ensure every person is treated as of equal worth. This moderation is of the sort the Moderator of the Presbyterian church uses where a concept of first amongst equals ensures the necessary moderation of the power of the professionals. His second moderator he refers to as "Meteorological", a sort of damping down, a maintaining of distance in relationship. Thus a professional may indeed love a patient but not as a relative, friend or lover does. Campbell would suggest that there is a vital detachment in the way a doctor loves a patient. This is a non-rational connection or reaching out from the doctor to the patient to truly appreciate and enhance the patient as a human being. The moderation inherent in the professional role maintains important boundaries.

Later Campbell talks about "the sacrament of care" which in medicine may reach a moment of very high reality in palliative care.

He suggests that "a caring response to someone who may soon die creates and discovers the value which cannot be destroyed. It refuses to discard the person because the organism is decaying. This is the secular sacrament of medical care".

There is a great kinship between the love that is implicit in this view and the statement by Dame Cicely Saunders that underpinned her attitude when setting up the modern hospice movement.

'You matter because you are you, and you matter until the last moment of your life.'

There is powerful undercurrent of love running through these different ways of valuing human beings which is very much part of the love I am trying to define in medicine.

Another aspect of medical love is its practicality. This love is not some sort of hand wringing, wishing the world was a better place and wanting everyone to be happy; that is an unhelpful, sentimental fluffy nonsense. This love found in medicine deals with the hard currency of blood, pain, vomit, incontinence, fear, delirium, delusion and death. It is very much about looking into the eyes of a person in despair at three in the morning and being prepared hold their gaze.

It is also about having specialised knowledge to help and knowing when to use, and when not to use, such knowledge. So, love in medicine exists on a foundation of competence, of learning, of continued study and reflection. It is a hard-won thing that needs continuous care. This love is not merely about wanting to give pain relief to a suffering person, it is about knowing their renal function as well as knowing why that matters. In *Letters to a Young Surgeon*, Richard Selzer cautions against making love in medicine a kind of self-indulgence and suggests it comes from repetitive acts of healing and care.

Then, he says, 'You will not announce your love but will store it up in the bodies of your patients to carry with them wherever they go.'

The National Health Service in the UK is the context that the vast bulk of medical encounters, and hence medical love, takes place. Another window giving a glimpse of love in medicine is provided by Ballatt and Campling in their fascinating book *Intelligent Kindness*. Here they suggest that the NHS encourages doctors and other healthcare workers to attend to the deep values of society. They suggest that there is a well of community and common interests that the NHS taps into. This is a clue as to why the NHS remains so popular with society at large, despite its many perceived shortcomings. Perhaps this is why even doctrinaire politicians of different parties realise that to question the value of the NHS is almost to question some of the fundamental values of society itself. Even if politicians do not consciously recognise where this very high regard for the NHS comes from, they are very wary indeed of being suspected by the electorate of not wholeheartedly believing in the NHS.

In this excellent and thought-provoking book, the authors develop wider arguments about the need to change the managerial and regulatory frameworks of the NHS to nurture rather than discourage such fundamental values and to encourage intelligent kindness. These arguments go beyond the scope of what I am looking at here, but they clearly spring from the same roots as medical love. This connection with deep common values of community and humanity, this intelligent kindness, is very much a part of love in medicine.

Iona Heath in her wonderful commentary on death and dying *Matters of Life and Death* illuminates an important aspect of love in medicine when she considers the role of general practitioners. Although love as such is not mentioned, I think that her consideration of the role of GPs clearly reflects love as I understand it as it is found in medicine, and has echoes of intelligent kindness too. Heath notes that GPs sometimes find it difficult that their work is not always understood by policy makers as well as they would hope because "… the sort of gentle, persistent, undramatic, science-based care at which general practitioners excel is only really valued by the sick, the vulnerable, the frightened and the frail".

This exemplifies much what I understand to be love in medicine and clearly shows how that love is manifest – in a supremely practical manner.

There are limits to this love and important caveats. Some people, such as Paul Bloom in his book *Against Empathy* have argued against too close an emotional involvement by the doctor in the therapeutic relationship. They emphasise the value of a certain detachment, a distance. Bloom makes this point well and it might be seen as an argument against love in medicine although he does not explicitly state this. His understanding of empathy involves the healthcare worker actually feeling and sharing the pain of their patient or client, and this clearly has the danger of placing an intolerable and unsustainable burden on the healthcare worker. How can anyone allow such endless suffering and pain into their souls without being overwhelmed?

Yet a different understanding of empathy involves the healthcare worker being aware of their patient's pain, of that pain mattering to them, then communicating that awareness and care to the patient. This is closer to my understanding of empathy and is also completely consistent with love in medicine. Indeed, it is one of the important ways that Campbell's moderators can operate on love to keep it within the boundaries necessary for professionalism and sustainability. Again, this is not the love that might exist in a family or between spouses for instance: it is moderated.

Love in medicine, as I have emphasised, is a practical matter very mindful of what can be done, how to help. Yet it also has a different aspect, where choosing not to do something is the best option. Doctors starting to learn about palliative medicine are advised that sometimes they should 'not just do something, sit there'.

The act of being with a patient without necessarily doing anything is of central importance, and is somewhere that I see love in medicine clearly manifest. In *Intoxicated by My Illness*, Broyard makes this point strongly. He notes:

'I see no reason or need for my doctor to love me – nor would I expect him to suffer with me… I just wish he would *brood* on my situation for perhaps five minutes, that he would give me his whole mind just once, be *bonded* with me for a brief space, survey my soul as well as my flesh, to get at my illness, for each man is ill in his own way.'

There is a paradox here as Broyard specifically does not want love from the doctor and yet I am arguing that love is essential in medicine. But if we accept the love as I have evolved the term thus far, and further we recognise Bloom's warning about his definition of empathy, then the paradox is resolved. Broyard is not asking for love as it is often considered; he does not want to be swept into the doctor's arms or for the doctor to completely share his pain, but he is simply asking to be really seen. He asks for the doctor to be truly present and to see him as a human being. He later elaborates on this theme when he says:

'I'd like my doctor to scan *me*, to grope for my spirit as well as my prostate. Without some such recognition I am nothing but my illness.'

To me Broyard is suggesting a clear manifestation of love by warning us to resist the subtle pressure that doctors can feel to reduce someone to nothing but their illness, reduce them to 'the gallbladder in bed four', or 'the stroke in casualty'.

Emotional granularity can help us with this vital ingredient of love in medicine. There is an indigenous Australian word "Dadirri" which means a deep, spiritual act of reflective and respectful listening. The same underlying power is present in dadirri as in Broyard's plea to be seen.

Both involve one human being paying rapt attention to another human being. The attention is conditional only upon it being an interaction between two human beings and in a therapeutic context it is a manifestation of love.

The last word on this should be left to that master of words who looked at medicine with such great clarity, the late Richard Selzer, poet and surgeon, in his masterpiece *Mortal Lessons*. He notes:

'I do not know when it was that I understood that it is precisely this hell in which we wage our lives that offers us the energy, the possibility to care for each other. A surgeon does not slip from his mother's womb with compassion smeared upon him like the drippings of his birth. It is much later that it comes. No easy shaft of grace this, but the cumulative murmuring of the numberless wounds he has dressed, the incisions he has made, all the sores and ulcers and cavities he has touched in order to heal. In the beginning it is barely audible, a whisper, as from many mouths. Slowly it gathers, rises from the streaming flesh until, at last, it is a pure *calling* – an exclusive sound, like the cry of certain solitary birds – telling that out of the resonance between the sick man and the one who tends him there may spring that profound courtesy the religious call love.'

Chapter 5
Spirituality

'It's when formal religion breaks down that spirituality is required.'

— Rabbi Lionel Blue, *My Affair with Christianity*

Before discussing spirituality and its fundamental importance to medicine, it helps to define it. This is where the first problem lies. Two international conferences on Medicine and Spirituality that I attended were wholly unable to agree any definition of spirituality. This was actually rather encouraging as it is an area where definitions and language can either break down or restrict things. Excepting those fundamentalists of different persuasions who saw the only place for 'true' spirituality to be wholly in their particular brand of religion or disbelief, most people agreed on it being a distinct entity with a greater or lesser overlap with religion.

Religion is pretty easily defined. Most definitions run something like this: a set of codified beliefs about the universe, often involving a supreme being or creator, with doctrine, sacred texts and forms of worship or devotion. Many people do of course see their own spirituality in terms of their religion even if they are open to possibility of spirituality being found in other places by people with different beliefs. There are, for instance, devout Christians I have met who would see spiritual insights in Islam or in Buddhism, and the other way round. Interfaith and belief fora are mutually enriching.

So here is one suggestion for a definition of spirituality which (of course!) leans heavily on many people much wiser than me.

'Spirituality can be thought of as the quest for meaning, especially in relation to that which is transcendent.'

This allows spirituality to exist entirely within religion, entirely out of religion or with varying degrees of overlap with religion or religions. But some people find, as I do, that the term "religious" is a monolithic term that can fail to do justice to the subtleties and complexity of individual experience. So this definition does also allow a variety of different interpretations of spirituality depending upon different viewpoints which consider aspects of spirituality as understood by individual people. It may also permit an individual's view of spirituality to evolve over time, just as mine has. This flexibility and plurality of spirituality is crucial to help make it a constructive encounter when spirituality bumps into medicine, as I see that it very often does.

Perhaps the moment of highest reality for medicine and spirituality is in the context of life changing or life limiting illness, especially as seen in Palliative Care.

The World Health Organisation discussion of Palliative Care makes the point that "palliative care improves the quality of life of patients and their families who are facing problems associated with life-threatening illness, whether physical, psychosocial or spiritual".

Palliative Care clearly and explicitly recognises the importance of spirituality and places it centre stage. Yet why does it matter, what is the impact of addressing spirituality in this context? What is big deal about spirituality in this context?

There is a subtle problem to address first before discussing the impact of spiritual distress, and therefore of attention to spirituality, in medicine. If we define spirituality too loosely or correlate it too much with mental health, then a circular argument is set up where better spiritual health is associated with better mental health. So although there is considerable work on the relationship between these two – Harold Koenig for instance has written very helpfully on this – it is important to be sure that spirituality is what I am talking about.

There are ways of measuring spirituality which try to be specific: an example would be the FACIT-Sp scale. I don't want to get into an extensive academic discussion about this, but it is fair to say that there is considerable evidence that meaningful effects on patients and doctors do exist. These include spiritual well-being having an association with decreased desire for hastened death, hopelessness and suicidal ideation. And people with terminal illness seem to show an increased spirituality as death approaches. Patients seem also to value the chance to discuss their spiritual needs and to trust physicians who ask about such matters. It is also clear that religious and spiritual beliefs influence patients' decisions about medical interventions from blood transfusion to pain relief.

Dame Cicely Saunders, founder of the modern hospice movement, showed the vital and practical importance of this when she coined the term 'Total Pain'. She noted how so often pain could not be controlled purely by pharmacological means and realised that the pain was being fuelled not just by physical factors but by other factors such as psychological, social and spiritual factors too. What could be more pressing, more practical and more central to a doctor's work than the control of pain in terminal disease? Saunders' observation is now widely accepted in palliative care and we know that a doctor working in this area who is not aware of all these aspects of pain is doing a grave disservice to their patients. So a person's spirituality is of direct relevance to a doctor's work.

As so often in medicine, this recognition of the spirituality of our patients is not a one-way process. When we honour spiritual needs in patients, it helps our spiritual health as well. Doctors are spiritual beings caring for other spiritual beings. Healthcare separated from spirituality is often recognised to be incomplete and we neglect that at our peril. There is a lot of evidence for serious mental health problems in doctors which are bad for us as a profession, and also bad for our patients. And of course, we also are all patients at some point in our lives.

We doctors are not a healthy bunch. There are various measures of this ill health that have been used and here are a few just to illustrate the point. Suicide is maybe the worst outcome imaginable and statistically a very hard end point. Doctors do badly in this amongst comparable professions with female doctors especially at risk. Burnout rates can be very high – 50% in some studies and depression is also a problem. The British Medical Association a few years ago suggested the total cost of training a general practitioner, for instance, to be around half a million pounds. So the fact that so many doctors choose to leave the profession early and the reasons for this are very important, even provoking discussion in mainstream media.

Medical humanities is a field which looks at medicine through a wide lens to include other disciplines not usually thought of as relevant to medicine. These include historical, literary, religious, psychological and artistic aspects. This contribution of the humanities has been looked at in medical students, measuring burnout risk and reduction in empathy another was a significant correlation between meaningful positive qualities in students; personal empathy, tolerance for ambiguity, wisdom, emotional appraisal, spatial skills and an inverse correlation with some components of burnout. So it is clear that this area matters, and is it not merely a fluffy, pleasant, optional extra.

And this is relevant to spirituality, the quest for meaning, which can be fed by all of these different aspects of humanity. This is as true for doctors as for anyone else. Once I began to think of spirituality as being relevant to medicine, I realised that it was all around me, woven into so many human interactions. It was extraordinarily helpful and liberating to realise both that spiritual matters were no longer the preserve of the religious and that there could be an extra dimension to my consultations. This in no way inhibited my role as a doctor: I still needed to know about the technical, science-based care that is generally thought of the function of medicine, but I could also ask questions that that allowed another level of understanding. Patients welcomed being asked if they were religious or spiritual, and discussing what they were afraid of or gave them joy, and what gave their lives meaning.

Sometimes this might allow understanding of hitherto puzzling issues such as reluctance to take analgesia or sleeping medication. Their model of spirituality might make them see virtue in suffering for instance, and that would give a powerful opening for helpful discussion. The fact that I was clearly interested in them as a person, not just a patient, was also important and welcomed. Never have I come across opposition to such (careful) questioning and even if a patient politely declined to discuss spirituality I was never made to feel as if I had somehow been improper or invasive. A devout atheist who I fell into discussion with as I sat by her deathbed told me:

'Oh no, I'm not spiritual at all. I'm just a grain of sand in the cycle of evolution.'

This statement, beautiful in its gentle certainty, seemed pretty spiritual to me. It did also allow her to tell me a little more about things that were important to her, and for me to really see her as a person.

This tells us something about the range of guises that doctors might bump into spirituality when with other human beings who at that time are patients. I have seen a spectrum of spiritual understandings when people are faced with life changing or life limiting events. This richness of understandings as people dance around the meaning of the human condition in their own particular way is truly beautiful and a privilege to see.

Sometimes it is readily identified, as in a priest I remember who was dying of metastatic cancer and asked in despair, 'Where does this all come from?'

He needed special care and the right kind of spiritual support from a non-judgemental priest who could sit with him in his doubt. It also helped us to see why anxiety and depression were actually a more difficult problem than we had realised. He wanted to spare us his doubt as he felt that might be a betrayal of his calling. This shows another aspect of spiritual distress that I have repeatedly seen – the need some people with serious medical problems feel to spare others from the doubt, turmoil and distress.

Conversely a patient's certainty in spiritual matters is also very important for a doctor to recognise, and potentially catastrophic for us to undermine, either purposefully (rarely; who but a religious or secular fundamentalist would do such a thing?) or, more commonly, by blunder. Recently a woman dying in a hospice provided a good example of this. When I broached the subject of spirituality she was cheerfully and politely insistent, saying, 'I have a very strong faith and don't want anyone trying to convert me thank you. It's very kind of you to bother but I don't need any help.'

Her faith was shared with her family who were around her and it was a pleasure to be able to say how glad I was that they she did have this and I had no intention of trying to "convert" her. Her spirituality, her model of the universe, was not mine and in other circumstances I might have been up for a good discussion about it, but not in this situation. She was content and certain of where she was going. There was also, as far as an outsider could tell, no coercion or pressure from the family or others of her belief which might have been stopping her exploring any doubts or uncertainty.

Proselytising or undermining someone's belief at the end of life is a dreadful thing to do and the exact opposite of attending to spiritual needs of patients. There is evidence that as people near death their existing faith may be enhanced, but that faith does not emerge without having a faith initially.

Spirituality may be expressed in other ways too: beauty, art, music, nature, gardening, family or humanity in broadest sense. To give people space for these things or signal that they are acknowledged and respected is part of the holistic care of patients.

The Royal College of Psychiatrists has a special interest group in Spirituality with 3,600 members – over 19% of the total college membership – and this demonstrates how mainstream the idea of understanding and respecting spirituality is. An admission clerking of a Palliative Care patient would be considered incomplete without a spiritual history, however brief. Yet we know that healthcare professionals are not always good at discussing spirituality and indeed can feel uncomfortable doing so.

'How do I discuss spirituality?'

'What do I do with the information?'

'That is the chaplain's job, I'm a doctor not a priest.'

These are fair points. Clearly there are different medical situations where spirituality is more or less important. At one end of the spectrum might be Palliative Care where a doctor cannot do their job properly without acknowledging this aspect of care. At the other end might be the suturing of a wound in the Emergency Department or administering an anaesthetic for a hernia repair. But even here there might be a frightened patient or someone where the apparently minor problem was part of a wider issue and where some acknowledgement of the spirituality of the patient was worthwhile.

Enquiring about spirituality can also allow a doctor insight into the cultural and ethnic heritage of a patient. This is precious as information about, say, funeral practices but also a way of allowing the doctor to see more of the entirety of the human being in their care, and for that human being to know that they have been really seen and heard. Resolution of conflict as far as is realistic may sometimes be an important aspect of spiritual care. This may be conflict with religion or with other people, family and friends. These conflicts may need help to at least be recognised and addressed even if complete resolution is impossible.

Ill health, life altering or life limiting illness can be a series of losses for patients and they may have to discard many precious things on this journey. They may well have to let go of dreams. Dreams of travel to a longed-for place, seeing grandchildren grow up, walking the Pennine Way, learning to play the piano or countless other things that have been at the forefront of their goals or unacknowledged in the background.

There is a great deal in Bernard Shaw's well-known suggestion that "there are two great tragedies in life. One is not to get your heart's desire. The other is to get it".

Addressing spiritual issues in our patients, and in ourselves too, is often not about uncovering difficulties and then dealing with them. When faced with someone who is in a "dark night of the soul" it may be futile to try to find solutions. Of course true depressive illnesses must be watched for and treated appropriately and aggressively, but sometimes it is disrespectful to try to gloss over a deep problem with some trite platitude or well-intentioned attempt to "cheer them up". A phrase I heard some years ago during a slightly drunken meal was so apposite that I wrote it down on a paper napkin and have used it ever since.

'Sometimes the best we can do for someone is to sit and stare into the darkness together.'

So if spiritual care is so important, how does a doctor incorporate it into their practice? Some years ago, there were a series of "Spiritual Competencies" published by a well-known organisation. Well-meant though these efforts were, they seemed very mechanistic and left brain. The idea of trying to teach these seemed to me, and to some others involved with spiritual care at the hospice I was working at, all rather dispiriting. It was good to see this area given importance but how to make the teaching of spirituality in healthcare generally and medicine specifically more, well spiritual, was unclear. Such an apparently fuzzy concept needed some structure, some hooks to hang the ideas on to make it coherent and workable.

Enter Margaret Holloway, Professor at Hull University, who produced a very helpful report in 2011 for the NHS on Spiritual Care at the End of Life: the whole report is well worth reading in its own right. For this purpose, I want to concentrate on her suggestion of a "Fellow Traveller" model of spiritual care in healthcare. She suggested four levels of engagement.

First – Joining: starting where the person is – that is everyone's business in healthcare. We should all be prepared at this level.

Second – Listening: sensitivity to spiritual matters and assessment of the significant of spiritual issues. Everyone's business up to a point.

Third – Understanding: Spiritual empathy – this for workers with understanding of their own spirituality.

Fourth – Interpreting: spiritual exploration – only workers with special training and in conjunction with religious and spiritual care advisors, for instance Priests or Imams.

This stepped approach with explicit limits on how much it is appropriate for people to engage is very important and liberating. No doctors need fear that they are expected to be a spiritual expert or to know answers and deal with things beyond their competence. All that is necessary is a readiness to ask about spiritual matters, a preparedness to listen and validate the patient's (or relative's) spirituality. They can refer on to another, perhaps more appropriate or specialised, person if necessary.

There are other excellent initiatives, such as Opening The Spiritual Gate, which aim to root spirituality in medical practice in a concrete and practical way. These also help to give people a structure and language for spiritual discussion with patients. I have seen different opening gambits which allow ways into discussion of spiritual matters. What seems important is to give individual practitioners a way of discussing these things that is comfortable to them without somehow imposing an agenda on the patient.

'Would you call yourself a religious or spiritual person, are those things important to you?'

'What gives you strength in this situation?'

'Is there anything that has given you meaning in life?'

Or even statements which allow people to respond as they wish can be helpful.

'Some people find that when they are facing serious illness, they find themselves asking questions about life and about meaning.'

I really like Elizabeth Kubler-Ross's work and her contribution to the care of people has been colossal. I especially like one of her thoughts about matters of the spirit:

'Spirituality is like love; there are no experts, there is no right way.'

One way that also sometimes allows insights and shared understanding is with a lightness of touch that even includes humour. I have been talking about serious matters; illness, life and death, incapacity and loss. These deserve to be taken seriously, but not always solemnly. We have to earn the right to use humour, to have demonstrated unequivocally that we have heard what the patient has said and respected it before any lightness is possible. But just sometimes it may allow the patient a little power over their situation, to allow them to get one back on the grim hand they have been dealt.

David Tacey, in his thoughtful work *The Spirituality Revolution* discusses the 'Spirituality Gap' "… the ever-present and persistent gap between patients who report that 'spirituality' is an important element of their personal identity, so of mental health, and doctors who have no way of entering, at least professionally or 'legitimately', into this spiritual language and terminology".

Thankfully, this is now less true than it was in 2004 when Tacey wrote, and spirituality is gradually becoming recognised as an integral part of the proper business of doctoring. All of us, patients and doctors, are the better for such recognition.

Chapter 6

Science

*'Science, however, purports to be uncovering such a reality. Its apparent value-free descriptions are assumed to deliver **the** truth… Yet this highly objective stance, this "view from nowhere", to use Nagel's phrase, is itself value laden.'*

– Ian McGilchrist

'We are going to be guided by the science.'

Writing in 2020 during the COVID-19 pandemic this phrase or ones like it I hear frequently from politicians: and very welcome it is too: it has not always been so and much avoidable suffering has resulted. Science has been described as the great gift of our civilisation to the world allowing extraordinary understanding simply impossible without it. The scientific method involves generating a hypothesis, creating an experiment to confirm or refute that hypothesis, ensuring the result is repeatable. It thus gradually refines our model of the universe and the rules that govern it. Most importantly science allows the prediction of events and consequences outside of immediate experience.

Doctors either study sciences at school, or convert to medicine from the arts by a rigorous course in science after leaving school. Medicine is firmly planted amongst the sciences and not the arts; it uses the scientific method and understanding as immensely powerful tools that have produced transformative wonders such as vaccination, anaesthesia and asepsis. No one can reasonably doubt the power and benefit of so much that has been achieved using this method. And if one is trying select a blood pressure treatment, decide on antibiotic resistance or control a pandemic, science must underpin medicine. Terrible things can, and do, happen if science is ignored or even perverted. The lives needlessly lost as result of Andrew Wakefield's lies about vaccination are testament to this.

So one might say that we must ensure the scrupulous application of science to medicine at all times, and that is pretty much all that needs to be said here. I understood this very early on in my medical career, helped considerably by a year studying zoology before switching to medicine. All that was required was the constant refining of our knowledge by the scientific method with the exposure of pseudo-science, and all would be well. Yes, I do still think that and still I consider science as a bedrock on which those of us who spend careers trying to help and comfort the sick can stand, and upon which so much of the edifice of medicine is built.

This way that a foundation of science can interplay seamlessly with the human spirit to produce something of great beauty is illustrated by Iona Heath in *Matters of Life and Death: Key Writings.*

Amongst many insights in this extraordinary book Heath laments the inability of politicians to see the value of General Practice in the UK. It is worth repeating in this context the quote of hers I referred to earlier that:

'Yet perhaps this is inevitable because the sort of gentle, persistent, undramatic, science-based care at which general practitioners excel is only really valued by the sick, the vulnerable, the frightened and the frail. In relatively prosperous countries these groups will always tend to be in a relatively easily marginalised minority.'

Clearly science and good medicine can co-exist very well.

But it is more complex than that. When helping to teach a Master's in Integrated Healthcare a few years ago I ended up designing and leading a module on different paradigms of healthcare. When I started looking into what we were going to cover, I expected to just illustrate the deficiencies of other healthcare approaches, and either look at them critically through my scientific lens or even dismiss them utterly as having no value compared with my approach. Sometimes that did indeed happen. But even using the standard scientific approach of controlled trials there is evidence that some apparently unscientific therapies can work, for some the evidence is inconclusive and some really are ineffective. A few have the potential for real harm.

But then some really interesting things started to happen as I looked into the scientific paradigm more carefully. First was the value of stepping back from the normal scientific model, as discussed a bit more in the chapter on healing. The second point was more interesting still: a realisation that science is not only more subjective than we think but also the limits to what the methodology can achieve. I was introduced to two thinkers – Thomas Kuhn, a famous philosopher of science who wrote *The Structure of Scientific Revolutions*, and the lesser known Ludwik Fleck, a physician whose book

Genesis and Development of a Scientific Fact is, if anything, even more interesting.

The gift that Kuhn and Fleck give to us is understanding of some of the limitations of science as we usually think of it. This in no way undermines the great power for good that science is to the world, but it begins to help us see where it fits in, where it helps.

An example of the power of the scientific method as used in medicine might be something like this: 'We have given this treatment to thousands of people with your condition and with similar characteristics to yours and it has reduced their chances of getting this particular complication, so we can predict that it will be likely to help you.'

This sort of prediction is of enormous benefit in many situations: prevention of strokes, vaccination, treatment of HIV, repair of aortic aneurysms and countless other situations. It is especially useful at population based, group-based questions. It is always a moot question as to how such group-based evidence can be applied to individual cases, but it is the best thing we have.

But Kuhn and Fleck show us how the questions we ask, the evidence we select to use, the facts that we see are actually far more subjective than we generally realise. Kuhn and Fleck help us to see where our knowledge sits in the world. This in turn helps us to ask better questions, and perhaps even see more clearly things that we are not expecting to see. Fleck's extraordinary insight is that we are all in "Thought Collectives" of people whose thought processes and underlying assumptions as to the nature of reality are the same as our own. We are unconsciously inhibited from seeing things differently and so we tend to see what expect to see.

Fleck notes that "the mood of the thought collective of natural science is further realised in a particular inclination to objectivise the thought structure that it has created… The disciplined, shared mood of scientific thought… yields the specialised thought style of science… whether the realisation of the thought style has been consistently achieved and in particular whether procedure has conformed to tradition (or preparatory training)… and convert what has been presented into scientific fact".

So Fleck shows us the danger of not realising that we are in some sort of echo chamber when immersed in science. I saw a perfect example of this when Rupert Sheldrake had presented some work on telepathy to a conference we were both addressing. He reported clear, well designed experiments showing that telepathy does indeed occur and that we can demonstrate the truth of this by repeating the experiments ourselves.

A physicist in the audience said how he was not prepared to listen to such unscientific nonsense that "just could not be true". Rupert's reply was that he could see three possibilities.

First: He, Rupert, was lying. But the evidence was on his website and the questioner could repeat the experiments himself.

Second: He had misinterpreted the results. But again, the evidence was there for everyone to check.

Third: Our model of the universe was incomplete.

None of this satisfied the questioner who remained wholly unconvinced.

I was struck by how profoundly unscientific the questioner had been. He was unconsciously so stuck in his thought collective that he could not apply any objective methodology to the data and had to reject it all out of hand because it was 'impossible'. And this from a physicist whose discipline routinely deals in all sorts of ideas that seem to outsiders like me wonderfully improbable: such as the results of experiments being affected by observing them, electrons only having a probability of existence in a particular place, time being relative and variable, and non-locality of events.

This recognition not only of the limits of our knowledge but also of our ways of acquiring knowledge can be very helpful when we come across patients or practitioners whose models of the world do not fit easily into our scientific medical model. This understanding can give us some protection against the hubris of dismissing something that our patients find works and to be useful just because to our model the evidence the patient tells us about seems "impossible". Fleck helps us to see that sometimes what seems to us impossible is in fact merely incongruent with our thought collective. Kuhn agrees, noting that "normal science, for example, often suppresses fundamental novelties because they are necessarily subversive of its basic commitments".

None of this is new. Antoine Lavoisier in the eighteenth century was a genius who made enormous contributions to chemistry and biology. He laid the foundations of the modern periodic table which is so fundamental to our modern chemistry. His eminence at the time was such that he was put in charge of a commission in France to investigate meteorites. He concluded that they were all fakes and had them removed from museums claiming that "the idea that rocks can fall from the sky is preposterous".

Even well-informed geniuses are caught in thought collectives and can be fallible. Max Planck notes drily that "a scientific truth does not triumph by convincing its opponents and making them see the light, but rather because its opponents eventually die and a new generation grows up that is familiar with it".

As science understands more about the universe there are some important limits worth considering. I am no mathematician, but have read a little about Kurt Godel, and his contribution to our understanding of the fundamental structures and forces of the universe. He showed that in mathematics there are theorems whose truth or falsehood cannot be proved. Some understand this to mean that there are limits to how much mathematics and science can be shown to explain the universe.

From the other side of the discussion about the limits of science I was fascinated to hear Jude Currivan talk about attempts to bring the macro level of physics (relativity) and the micro level (quantum mechanics) together in a coherent way. She has also written in more detail about this in *The Cosmic Hologram*. Her well-informed contention – Jude was a theoretical physicist to postgraduate level before going into business – is that theoretical physics is starting to paint a picture of the fundamental structure of the universe which has close parallels with long standing spiritual traditions. This may also be giving clues as to how phenomena which many of us recognise as real but which do not fit into our normal model of the universe, such as healing for example, may actually turn out to have a theoretical underpinning.

So, to return to the sort of science that we normally consider shapes our usual medical understanding, it helps to consider what we as doctors might consider as evidence.

There is a sort of hierarchy of evidence that most scientists broadly agree with, and that it is rarely questioned.

The gold medal goes to Meta-Analysis of Randomised Controlled Trials (RCTs). RCTs match two groups of patients and give one the treatment and the other no treatment (preferably 'blinded', where the patients do not know which treatment they are getting until the end of the experiment) and then the result observed. Ideally the trials are 'double blind', where the researchers themselves do not know who gets which treatment until afterwards. Meta-analysis is rigorous method whereby the information from many RCTs is combined systematically to give as reliable an answer as possible.

The Silver medal goes to individual RCTs with the proviso that an individual study can still get things wrong and 'significance' statistically still allows a one in twenty probability that the result is due to chance.

Only a Bronze medal is awarded to observational studies where something is tried on a particular group and the effect watched carefully.

Making the final, but out of the medals, are Qualitative studies where information about much subtler changes and things people say or feel about the subject under investigation is gathered and analysed very carefully. In fact, there are plenty of subjects well worth investigating where Qualitative research is the only possible way to look at things, and there are rigorous ways of analysing the data from these studies. People's attitudes to how doctors' break bad news to them, or asking what things they think are important in how a hospital is being run, would be good examples. In fact, qualitative research can give priceless information about matters where the quantitative methods so widely lauded must remain silent.

Not even making the final are Anecdotal Reports. One-off statements about individual cases. Rarely much help for research in themselves they can help generate questions to consider with other, better, methods. And yet these can just occasionally be very influential when doctors discuss cases – perhaps at times too influential as we are creatures that like stories. But sometime the anecdotal report is all we have.

So meta-analysis of RCTs is considered the gold standard of evidence in medicine. So much in fact that I remember admiring the senior doctor who, when presented with a possible treatment, just asked if there was a randomised double blind controlled study that proved that it worked: if there was not, he merely shrugged dismissively and that was that. Indeed, RCTs are excellent tools to decide questions such as which of two medications lowers blood pressure best or whether a new drug really helps cure peptic ulcers.

What they are not as good at is looking at how useful complex interventions with a number of variables might be, or how good treatments might be that are used in real life clinical situations rather than in clinical trials. Trying to see how helpful homeopathy is for instance, where it is not just the remedy prescribed that is the mainstay of the treatment but a whole lengthy consultation with a detailed history and (perhaps most significantly) a narrative or model of their illness that the patient has negotiated, understood, and accepted.

Paul Dieppe and others have suggested that for complex interventions RCTs might actually be less rigorous and less appropriate than other methodologies. These other methods might ask better questions that are more helpful in the real world. Randomised pragmatic designs and randomised cluster designs for instance might indeed be better than RCTs in particular situations. A detailed review of research methodology is outside the scope of this discussion but the point stands – sometimes what we think of as rigorous science is less objective and rigorous than we think.

To be clear: I have no time for pseudo-science, and the distrust of both science and expert opinion found in some quarters (the anti-vaccine lobby, for instance) is dangerous nonsense. Indeed, I am arguing here for recognising what science is good at (and it is really, really good at a lot of things) and knowing how to ask the correct questions of it. And we need to recognise when we are in a thought collective and the power that has to influence our thinking, for good and ill.

Evidence Based Medicine (EBM) is a very helpful way of encouraging doctors to use the best evidence available to treat individual patients. EBM tries explicitly to integrate clinical experience and the values and situation of the patient with the research about the problem being addressed. There are recognised sources of evidence available and, as in so many areas, the problem is not so much a lack of information – there is almost limitless information available on everyone's phone – but discernment about what is of value and what to do with it. The explicit point about integration of clinical experience and the patient's values being central to this process, is vital.

What is the function of evidence? This a disarmingly simple question, but one perhaps not asked often enough. In medicine, as in other branches of knowledge, evidence might be asked to do different things, to answer different questions.

In medicine we are generally asking evidence to guide us as to what we should do, or as importantly should not do, in a given situation. There might need to be quite different sorts of evidence depending upon which questions we are asking. There is a danger of spurious certainty if we ask the wrong questions of the data. The reduction in a certain risk from a particular trial population over a set time might not translate so exactly into a more general population over a longer period in a different setting.

The National Institute for Health and Care Excellence (NICE) might use one reliable sort of evidence – meta-analysis of published RCTs – to make a decision about which anti-hypertensive drugs to use in a particular patient group for instance. But even then, there will need to some subjective element which reflects cost considerations – there are, and always will be, only limited resources. Often NICE use fixed thresholds of cost per Quality Adjusted Life Year (QALY) saved. Even the way in which QALYs are decided will involve some subjective assessments of quality of life – a notoriously difficult and subjective subject, and at times very difficult ethical questions. To their great credit, whether one approves of the decision or not, NICE are very open about the ways in which they arrive at their decisions.

A quite different sort of evidence might be needed when a general practitioner is trying to decide whether to recommend a particular psychotherapist to their patient whose condition they have come to know well. The evidence in terms of controlled trials will help a little here although the current fixation with Cognitive Behavioural Therapy (CBT) for a limited number of sessions which is suggested by the NHS is not supported by as robust evidence as often hoped.

Yet there will be other factors the GP has to consider. What about this person sitting in front of me, what sort of person are they and what will appeal to them and motivate them? What experience have I had with the local therapists, what is the waiting list, can they pay, what time scale might they be up for, what has been tried already? A different set of questions are being asked, quite rightly, of a different sort of evidence.

Anrzej Szczezelik, professor of medicine in Cracow, has written in some detail about the influence of the humanities in medicine in his fascinating book *Catharsis: On the Art of Medicine*. One of the most helpful parts is when he discusses science:

'Science is not able to answer questions that start with Why? or What for? Questions asking about reality at its deepest level. It can reply only to questions beginning with How? A fact worth remembering when science pervades every area of human life, including the spiritual. Along with technology it has become the new religion.'

Even though as I have hinted earlier, spirituality and science might in the end turn out to be closer bedfellows than we currently accept, I think Szczezelik makes a very helpful point. This is a pertinent warning about the limits of science and the questions we should ask of it. A good servant but a bad master. I'll give the last word to that excellent humanist philosopher, Julian Baggini, who observes that "it is simply irrational to be too scientific about the human condition".

Chapter 7

Death

'When a man lies dying, he does not die from illness alone – he dies from his whole life.'

– Charles Peguy, *Basic Verities*

All doctors end up having more experience of dying, death, the dead, and the bereaved than most people. Your first dead body: maybe the one dissected as you try to learn anatomy while keeping the implications, the living and loving human being whose ruins you are searching through for knowledge, at arm's length. Some medical schools have dispensed with this ritual of dissection of bodies, but their first death will still not be long coming to a student. Maybe on a hospital ward, in general practice, or the emergency department: perhaps a total stranger or maybe someone you met as a living patient, laughed or talked with them before having to see them certified dead. The banality of the paperwork, the faces of the bereaved, the ultimate loneliness of those with no one left to grieve for them. Always the faint question at back of any doctor's mind or haunting the edge of their darkest dreams.

'Might I or my colleagues have done any more, postponed this a little, prepared the patient or others better: did I make any mistakes, could we have done better?'

Funny business, death. We can be utterly certain that it is waiting for us somewhere but not many people talk freely about it. A couple of centuries ago witnessing death was a commonplace. People died at home, perinatal and infant mortality was at levels we would find shocking today and children would have seen dead bodies aplenty. Now death often occurs in hospitals or other institutions away from home. It has become a medicalised process and yet paradoxically often considered a medical failure, as if we could keep death at bay for ever by the exercise of enough medical power. Iona Heath quotes Keizer in a telling comment on this.

'One of the most ill-starred meetings in modern medicine is that between a frail, defenceless old man nearing the end of his life, and an agile young intern at the beginning of his career.'

This medicalisation contrasts very starkly with the medieval view of death. For sure, many poorer people then just got on with life and death as best they could in terrible conditions, and utterly at the mercy of climate, harvests, war, and extreme social division. But there was still a widespread view that dying well, the "Ars Moriendi", was a moral activity. This involved active decisions by the dying person turning from the earthly preoccupations to contemplation of, and submission to, the divine. Belief in God, at least professed belief, was almost universal and the church wielded terrifying power. Priests, not doctors, were the key.

Now things could not be more different. Atul Gawande in his astute and excellent book *Being Mortal* seizes the current situation perfectly. He describes being the surgeon for a woman with a long story of bowel obstruction, rupture, sepsis, renal failure, heart attack, intensive care, ventilation, dialysis, gangrene, respiratory failure, intravenous feeding, and a leaking abdominal wound that might eventually heal, but only slowly. Gawande goes to talk with the family about a proposed tracheostomy and amputation. Her next of kin asks.

'Is she dying?'

Gawande writes.

'I did not know how to answer the question. I wasn't even sure what the word meant any more. In the past few decades medical science has rendered obsolete centuries of experience, tradition and language about our mortality and created a new difficulty for mankind: how to die.'

And the spiritual and religious background is very much part of all this change in how we view death. There are significant numbers of people for whom their religion gives clear guidance and clear answers, although even then there can room for doubt in particular circumstances, such as brain death or switching off ventilators for instance. For many people there are no clear frameworks from religion, and David Tacey in *The Spirituality Revolution* captures this well when he quotes Peter, one of his students.

'Like so many of my generation, I have had to walk among the ruins of what was once a stable, mighty spiritual empire; an empire that took millennia to build and only a few hundred years to collapse.'

I guess my personal journey with death and the dying has reflected a route taken by many doctors. From the terror of a newly qualified doctor thinking what I might have done wrong and wondering how much might I be blamed for this death, I have gradually become more at ease with the inescapability of death and recognising that death is rarely someone's fault or due to incompetence. Especially in the second part of my career, in palliative care, I have come to see the preciousness of helping someone have a good death. As we are all going to die, it matters.

What makes a good death? This is a fair question and also sheds light on what makes a bad death. Cardinal Basil Hume, when principal of Ampleforth School, suggested that his job was to prepare his pupils for death. And a good starting point is preparation for death. Montaigne says, '… We do not know where death awaits us: so let us wait for it everywhere. To practice death is to practice freedom.'

Starting to talk about death, what you want and do not want, is crucial and doctors often are well placed to help with these discussions. Similar themes keep coming up when people are asked to think about what would make a good death for them or for people they are close to. Freedom from pain or other physical symptoms such vomiting or breathlessness, in a setting of their choosing, surrounded by people who are close to them, with their affairs in order, at peace with their God or faith or belief, not being kept alive 'like a cabbage', not being a burden on other people and keeping as much dignity as possible. Pretty much the exact converse of these is what most people would consider a bad death.

Having the chance to talk about this with people who are up for the discussion, including perhaps a trusted doctor, is very important. It is our job to have ways to talk with people about the planning for the end of life and to encourage them to talk with the people they love. Such discussions can produce very helpful plans, sometimes formalised in a Living Will (a general non-binding discussion of wishes) or an Advance Decision to Refuse Treatment (legally binding and with real power).

I have learnt just how valuable such plans are, but also how difficult it is to make plans for the person you will become, in unknowable circumstances at some indeterminate time in the future. As Mike Tyson famously remarked:

'Everybody got plans until they get punched in the mouth.'

Yet this in no way invalidates the process or means such discussions are a waste of time – far from it. Certainly the most important result of advance care plans are the conversations that are triggered as a result; conversations much, much more important than any piece of paper.

When it comes to making plans, or better still the priceless discussions that result from the attempts to make plans, we naturally tend to think of the relatively predictable situation of an advanced cancer diagnosis, with a reasonably well understood disease process and subsequent decline. While that situation is important there are a couple of other categories that are maybe especially important. First there are the situations where people are living with illnesses that might kill them at any time though an exacerbation, like chronic obstructive pulmonary disease, but where aggressive hospital treatment can often return them to nearly (but generally not quite) where they were before.

Second there are cases with a very slow but inexorable decline, like dementia or even old age. Here there might be an insidious need for decisions about treatment that ideally should have been taken some time before. But by the time is obvious that a decision is necessary (about intensive care or attempted resuscitation for instance) it is often too late for rational discussion. The only way to help with these situations, most especially the slow death of dementia, must all discuss these things with those close to us at all stages of our lives: and keep discussing them.

An old couple I attended lived in a really well-run old people's home in one of the local villages. They had been devoted to one another, but as different diseases (Alzheimer's in one, multi-infarct dementia in the other) gradually robbed their brains of the capacity to be themselves, they were cared for in separate rooms. After some time, they both needed all care, could not recognise anyone or communicate in any way, seemingly oblivious to the world. They were thus for a year or more until the husband had another stroke that fatally damaged the part of his brain still keeping the autopilot going and he died. Perhaps it was just coincidence but a few days later his wife also died, of no particular crisis: she just packed up. Not for the first time, I was made to wonder about the levels of connection human beings have with one another.

Fear of death is certainly a major factor in any discussion. Philosophers from Epicurus to Nagel and Scheffler discuss why we are afraid of death and why we either should, or should not, fear death. This is all interesting and helpful. But the terms of the discussion and the questions, largely a matter of the intellect, necessarily frame the answers in terms of the intellect also. There is however another way of framing the discussion, in terms of evolution, which is not often considered and I think should be.

Humans are the current product of an unimaginably long period of Darwinian evolution, during which time our ancestors would have been subject to constant selection pressure to stay alive. Such a powerful and relentless desire not to die would have stood them in good stead through the famines, droughts, climate change catastrophes, incessant predation and other terrors that our ancestors were subject to. A group of humanoids who were relaxed in the face of imminent death would ultimately have survived – and bred – less than another group who were driven by the terror of personal extinction to fight to the bitter end. We are now, rightly, concerned about the sorts of death that we may face, but in the distant past our ancestors would have faced, and witnessed, an appalling litany of painful and violent deaths. This evolutionary, atavistic, legacy of humans to fear and oppose death needs to be understood and acknowledged if we are to help people die good deaths.

This means doctors have to accept the visceral and irrational nature of our fear. We must talk and listen to patients and make plans, that is certain, and although spiritual or religious support is vital it may not alone be enough. It can seem odd to an observer that a deeply religious person who believes they are going to heaven after they die is still terrified of death. It is part of a doctor's job to give a patient permission to say if they are frightened and reassurance that it may not be a lack of faith that makes them so, but that it is an inescapable part of the human condition.

We must recognise the frightened ancestral humanoid still cowering in the dusty recesses of our DNA. Appropriate physical touch, emotional connection and early demonstration of (for instance) the ability to control pain will all help here.

People facing death may find great comfort in the demonstration that pain can be controlled and they may well choose not to use that pain relief as much thereafter just knowing that they have it available.

There is an important distinction between fear of death, and fear of dying. Often when I had the chance to really talk with patients about fear of death, it was not the actual being dead that bothered them so much as the process of dying. They might assume that dying of cancer, for instance, was always terribly painful and the only way of avoiding that was either being dosed up with drugs to the point of unconsciousness or to have what has now become known as Assisted Dying (euthanasia or physician assisted suicide). So careful and honest discussions about what is possible with proper palliative care can be very useful to genuinely give people options at the end of their lives.

But I have learnt to heed another of Iona Heath's warnings that "the ambition that medical care should enable people to die 'symptom-free' seems to me an unattainable and dangerously dishonest chimera".

Such an honest discussion, including about the trade-offs between medications and side effects, will make it clear that dying will involve suffering to some degree. One inescapable source of suffering is simply the grief inherent in the dying experience with the impending loss of those they love and who they will leave behind when they die. But people of any faith or none may still find it helpful to remember one of the main things that the Buddha taught, that suffering is an inescapable part of life as well as of death.

The grief and bereavement of gradual losses, the possibility of physical suffering and the loss of control of one's destiny that is inherent in dying can lead people to believe that a sudden and unexpected death is much better all around.

'I just want to conk out. Wake up dead one morning.'

This initially an attractive sounding option, but from what I have seen, this may not always be best for everyone. There seem to be two problems with a sudden and unexpected death. Obviously, we cannot ask the person who has died suddenly what they think of it. But talking to people who have known that they were dying and had the chance to prepare for their death, they often seem to think of that as a very precious time and are glad that they had it. I have even heard people talk about this time as a precious gift. There is the chance to set things in order, make peace with people, say the things you want to say. And for those left behind the sudden death may be very traumatic with no chance for them to say goodbye or to prepare in any way. Especially hard can be cases where someone has terminal illness and everyone is expecting death to be weeks or months away, but then the person dies suddenly and wholly unexpectedly. This can be especially hard for the people left behind.

Part of this process of a person preparing for death may involve them looking back over their life. This can be a formal life review where there is a systematic attempt to deal with unresolved conflict and to be at peace with approaching dissolution of the self in death. But life review may be just an informal recognition of the wholeness of a person, that includes the person they were, as well as the person they now are as they are dying. The great psychologist Erikson suggested that the task in the eighth and last stage of life, as he had defined it, was to resolve integrity versus despair. He saw this task as involving acceptance of one's life choices, the road travelled and thus having no fear of death. He also suggested that there might be maladaptive and malignant results from not succeeding at this task: not accepting the advancing of years producing disgust and contempt for one's own and others' life with anger and despair.

It may not necessarily be a doctor's responsibility to help the dying to resolve these issues but I have come to realise that I should certainly be aware of the importance of such process and provide guidance about to who might help. I also deeply appreciate the chance to know something more of the dying person who I am attending as their doctor. Realising that the frail old man in the bed once led twenty men ashore at the Dieppe landings, and then led only one survivor back, was an important part of caring for him as a person.

We seem acutely aware of the moment of death, of its timing, and doctors are always asked, 'How long will it be?' and 'Has she died?' These universal questions, apparently so simple and reasonable are in fact difficult. The evidence shows that doctors are pretty useless at estimating how long someone with a terminal illness has to live. And when we do give an estimate people often die sooner than we predict. This despite the stories one hears about 'the doctors only gave him six months but he was still going strong a year later'. So I have learnt to be careful and vague. It may not be what the patient or the family want, but at least it is honest and in the end less harmful not to give spuriously exact predictions.

The moment of death has to determined, for legal and administrative reasons if for nothing else. But so often one is dealing with a process and not a moment. I have grown to see wisdom in the Buddhist idea of just leaving the body undisturbed for a while after death has apparently occurred, in order for the spirit to depart. Watching my mother-in-law dying was a great privilege. We had sat with her for an hour or more, then over about 20 minutes she gently left. There was a moment when we noticed no more breathing and slowly the life force visibly left her to leave an empty shell. It was clear that her body was then empty of the life that had been there for over ninety years. We had to give a time of death of course, but it was really rather arbitrary.

As so often, Richard Selzer, the master of words and medicine, sums this up so well in *Mortal Lessons*.

'You do not die all at once. Some tissues live on for minutes, even hours, giving their little cellular shrieks, molecular echoes of the agony of the whole corpus. Here and there a spray of nerves dances on. True, the heart stops; the blood no longer courses; the electricity of the brain sputters, then shuts down. Death is now *pronounceable.* But there are outposts where clusters of cells yet shine, besieged, little lights blinking in the advancing darkness. Doomed soldiers they battle on. Until Death has secured the premises all to itself.'

What happened often, so often in fact that I would routinely warn relatives about it, was that in a curious way people seemed to choose to die alone. Far more often than by chance, even when relatives or friends kept a bedside vigil for days on end, when the patient was alone whilst the relatives went to have a coffee or whatever for a few minutes, the patient 'chose' that moment to die. If they are not warned, people can think that they have failed, that they have abandoned their loved one at such an important time. Very often people have promised never to leave the person who is dying. This needs careful handling and reframing of what the promises they made mean, and suggesting that this is absolutely not abandoning their loved one. In reality it is true to say that the relatives love the person so much they have given them the chance to die alone if that is what they need. Even people deeply unconscious for days did this: not always, of course, but often enough for it to be both normal and still extraordinary at the same time.

And it also sometimes seems to help the deeply unconscious person to be told by those close to them that it is OK to die now. They can say how much they love them, will miss them but that they will be OK, and if it is time to go, then they must go. This clearly can help those left behind and oddly too it seems to allow people to die who have been hanging on in some odd way. What is going on there, how does it work? I have no idea.

Another aspect of death that I have continued to bump into is that of The Afterlife. For some that is a relatively straightforward concept. The atheist is clear that this life is all there is: after death, oblivion. And there is often much peace in that certainty. As one humanist atheist put it to me.

'I was fine for the untold billions of years the universe existed before I was born so I'll be fine for the untold billions after I die.'

There is therefore no worry about judgement, and consequently they have no truck with people trying to "save them".

Equally those with a strong faith, devout Christians for example, even if tested by a dark night of the soul when ill, may have real joy at the thought of being welcomed by a loving, just, and forgiving God with the words.

'Well done, my good and faithful servant.'

Certainly their fellow believers can take great comfort in their grief from the knowledge that they will meet their loved one again in Heaven. And other religions too with their clarity of belief can give similar help to the dying and to the bereaved. This can very occasionally be a barrier to openness, with both relatives and patient feeling they must each not let the other down by voicing any doubt. This is something we must acknowledge. But if I do seriously suspect this, then tiptoeing carefully between sowing seeds of doubt (a terrible crime against the dying) and allowing space for the patient to voice any doubts they might have, is hard but crucial.

'Afterlife' can mean something else altogether. The modern-day philosopher Samuel Scheffler has drawn attention to this in his ground breaking book *Death and the Afterlife*. Scheffler uses the term Afterlife to mean that which we leave behind after our lives have ended. This can be considered as a 'Collective Afterlife' where humanity and those around us continue to exist and to matter long after we are gone. This continuation is very important to us, perhaps under some circumstances it is more important than the continuation of our own lives. By various thought experiments Scheffler explores this idea and it is clear that this really matters. So the dying value this form of Afterlife greatly. This is both on a personal level – family, friends, work and a species or global level – the continuation and well-being of humanity and the world. A doctor who wishes to give good care to people dying in her or his care at least needs to acknowledge this area of possible concern.

I earlier alluded to Assisted Dying (AD) and one of the drivers for this being the desire for control, and fear of terrible things at the end of life. This is an issue which cuts across many boundaries of religion, belief, ethics, and profession. There are thoughtful, ethical, compassionate and well-informed people on both sides of this debate. The balance of my own belief is that the legalisation of AD in the UK would cause more harm than good. But this also means I do not think that I can deal here with this issue adequately or in a balanced way, doing justice to both sides of the debate. The issue is more complex and demands more careful thought than many people acknowledge. So the only further point I will make about AD is a commentary on a video of a case of euthanasia in Holland. The palpably good and caring doctor carried out the procedure entirely properly according to the regulations and law in Holland. The patient had fairly advanced motor neurone disease (MND) and he clearly wanted to die by euthanasia, trusting in his doctor. One of the reasons the patient gave for his decision was that he did not want to choke to death and he believed this was a big risk. But a careful prospective study of 112 MND patients showed none who died of choking and 88% dying peacefully. So there are many important points to be debated and I am by no means certain I am correct in being against AD, but it is vital that such a debate is well informed.

'The Granite Quality of Death' was an expression I was introduced to a while ago. It meant that the reality of imminent death in oneself or in others is so uncompromising, so immovable and so implacable that it had the effect of either smashing or least questioning many very basic assumptions we make. So we normally get on with our lives without questioning too much, concentrating on the myriad distractions and burdens of life until death appears, as it always does in the end, to jolt us into questioning and addressing things we have managed conveniently to ignore until then. And in many ways that is understandable – life has to go on after all. But even if we take Montaigne's advice to have nothing in mind more than death, to be familiar with it: the reality of death actually being present is different. And doctors need to remember that our patients with life limiting illness, and their relatives, have just crashed into that granite.

There is another very special role we as doctors play in death. This is the role of the compassionate observer: a role our colleagues a century or two ago would have understood well yet which is not so comfortable for a much more interventionist profession today. When our patients are dying this is the role of 'the familiar of death'. John Berger in his masterpiece *A Fortunate Man* explains.

'The doctor is the familiar of death. When we call for a doctor, we are asking him to cure us and to relieve our suffering, but if he cannot cure us, we are also asking him to witness our dying. The value of the witness is that he has seen so many others die… he is the living intermediary between us and the multitudinous dead. He belongs to us and he has belonged to them. And the hard but real comfort which they offer through him is still that of fraternity.'

The use for the word 'familiar' here as a noun reflects both the usual use (one who is familiar with, accustomed to) and the medieval use where the familiar was a spirit in physical form who connected mortals with another world. Broyard in *Intoxicated by My Illness* makes a similar point when he discusses the role of a doctor when a patient is dying.

'… So the doctor must usher the patient out of the world… the doctor is the patient's only familiar in a foreign country.'

Chapter 8
Humanities and Dignity

'Buddhism and monotheism, the religious and the secular, science and art, literature and myth. In exploring the fertile spaces between traditions, we open up a path that may be rooted in a specific tradition but has branched out into the no-man's-land between them all.'

– Stephen Batchelor, *Living with the Devil*

Many medical students become so fully occupied with trying to cram enough facts into their heads to get through the inevitable exams that stand between them and being a doctor, that a great deal that is not directly relevant to passing those exams gets elbowed out. Medical schools in the UK are currently making genuine attempts to remedy this: as an example Exeter Medical School has a series of mandatory Special Study Units in subjects either partly or wholly outside medicine. The discipline of medical humanities with its interdisciplinary involvement of the humanities, social science and the arts does have influence. This enlightened and very welcome.

But there is still a feeling that such studies are somehow a pleasant extra, nice enough if one has the time, but not the real business of medicine.

'When I am seriously ill, I want a doctor who can sort out my electrolytes rather than discuss poetry or the latest addition to the National Gallery.'

I remember this remark by a senior doctor over forty years ago, and at the time it seemed a hard argument to counter, although in retrospect I realise that the remark was made more to provoke discussion than as a serious attempt to devalue medical humanities. Nonetheless this doctor was making an important point which deserved an answer then and still deserves an answer now. If the choice we have to make, as implied by the remark, is indeed between a mastery of the complexities of technological medicine or a wider appreciation of those varied things that enrich us as human beings – then who would argue that doctors must choose the technological mastery?

At the time of hearing that remark as a medical student, despite being uneasy about it, I was unable to mount a coherent argument against that sentiment. But over my medical career I have become much clearer that not only do I disagree, but that the question itself I have come to recognise as one of the "When did you stop beating your wife?" sort. The whole terms of the question are wrong and to answer the question as it stands is to implicitly accept a false underlying premise. Once this category of questions was pointed out to me a few years ago, it is surprising how often they crop up. We regularly see reporters and interviewers in the media using this technique to steer the interview in a particular direction.

No one could rationally argue against the idea that doctors need high levels of technological competence, team working, problem solving, pattern recognition and ability to sift through and order vast amounts of data. We also need resilience and confidence to cope with high pressure, with uncertainty and with managing risk. Medical schools specifically look for these abilities in prospective doctors and nurture them throughout training. Training itself is recognised to be a continuing process throughout a doctor's career. So maybe literature and the humanities should be confined to just our free time, just to the margins and considered at best a pleasant enough optional extra and at worst a distraction from the real business of medicine?

I have heard some people grumbling about the overloading of doctors' minds, already with so much to learn, with all of this useless stuff like poetry, literature, the arts. Curiously, there is a helpful illustration from literature itself which encapsulates all that is wrong with this argument. Arthur Conan Doyle, himself a medical doctor as well as an author, introduces us to his great fictional detective Sherlock Holmes in *A Study in Scarlet*. Conan Doyle has Holmes observe that "… a man's brain originally is like a little empty attic… A fool takes in all the lumber of every sort… knowledge which might be useful to him gets crowded out… skilful workman is very careful indeed as to what he takes into his brain… nothing but the tools which may help him in doing his work… a mistake to think that that little room has elastic walls and can distend to any extent".

If this is indeed the case, then I, and those who believe in the humanities as essential in medicine have lost the argument.

But the fictional Holmes, for all his alleged brilliance and the actual brilliance of his author, has given us a wholly misleading analogy. In fact, the brain is better considered a muscle: the more it is used then the better it works and indeed the more varied ways it is used the more flexible and useful it is. Is a doctor who has an interest outside medicine – be it music, painting, history of London Rivers, flying jet aircraft to name but a few real examples – any less good at their primary work? Actors note that learning lines for a play becomes easier the more they do it. The idea of finite space and crowding out of important knowledge is simplistic and wrong.

The view that there is a binary choice between either appreciation of the humanities or medical excellence is therefore profoundly mistaken: it is not an either/or situation. Doctors are indeed expected to be doctors not artists or writers or composers, and rightly so: yet I have become sure that there is a strong case for encouraging and nurturing the humanities, literature and the arts in medical practice. And while there might inevitably be some retaining of new information, even learning of literature and poetry or acquisition of related skills, this is by no means essential to the understanding and appreciation of the humanities, or to being nourished by them. I believe that this wider understanding of the human condition is not merely desirable for doctors, but indispensable.

Humans like telling and hearing stories – stories help us to make sense of the world. We can be thought of as hard wired for stories. It is striking how an individual story can be much more powerful to the listener or the reader than any amount of carefully rehearsed argument. The media, and those who are expert at using the media, know this well. One picture of a patient with a good story can be much more powerful than a mountain of data or controlled trials when it comes to swaying public opinion. That may not be a good thing, but it is the case.

So what of fiction, imaginary stories, and their place in medicine? Good fiction contains truth that we recognise. I cannot improve on Stephen King's suggestion that "fiction is a lie, and good fiction is the truth inside that lie".

This is true in literature influencing the practice of medicine as well. There are truths, insights and benefits which I do not believe can be found as richly in medicine considered purely as a science as they are found in literature.

Palliative care, where cure is no longer possible and where the best we can do as doctors is to ease symptoms and provide comfort, is an area where I have seen how precious the insights and perspective of literature can be. The clearest example of palliative care being enriched by literature comes from the pen of that master observer and chronicler of the human condition, Leo Tolstoy. *The Death of Ivan Illych* is extraordinary. All those who have dealings with the dying would benefit from reading this relatively short novel. And all those who do so will see Tolstoy's clarity of observation not only of the external process of someone learning that they are dying, but also their inner world.

I have seen a slightly abridged version of this read out as a lecture in just under an hour, with thought provoking slides illustrating contemporary resonances. I have also read it myself to colleagues, including medical students. People are spellbound by the way in which Tolstoy so carefully notes Illych's journey, suffering and redemption. It would be rare for a Palliative care clinician, dealing with the dying every working day, not to gain considerably from this pocket masterpiece of literature. The depth of Tolstoy's insight is shown by the way in which Illych begins to feel isolated by the difficulty his family, friends and colleagues have in being honest with him. He colludes with this and thereby increases his own despair and misery knowing this to be so even as he does it.

'Ivan Illych's great misery was due to the deception that for some reason or other everyone kept up with him – that he was simply ill, not dying, and that he need only keep quiet and follow the doctor's orders, and then some great change for the better would be the result... made miserable by their persisting in lying over him about his awful position, and in forcing him too to take part in this lie.'

Tolstoy's description of the psychological element of physical pain cannot be bettered. But then Tolstoy includes the character of Gerasim, the servant, who alone knows how to treat him with honesty, who will look unflinchingly at his suffering and physical degradation and still see him. This is of immense comfort to him, more than the doctor's opium which is given with a lie.

As well as a knowing what needs to be done with medications, investigation and interventions, so much of what a doctor brings to a consultation with someone who is dying is just themselves. The open and compassionate witnessing of a human being, being ready to acknowledge the truth about the situation in the exactly the way that the fictional Ivan Illych needed and showed us so powerfully is paramount.

Yet it is far from just palliative care that needs these wider views from outside medicine. All fields of medicine can benefit from this, all doctors can have their souls nurtured by the humanities. Surgery, despite being a very wide and varied field in itself, is not the first place that we might think of literature, poetry and the humanities having a place. Yet part of the brilliance of Richard Selzer is to root his specialty of surgery so firmly in reflective literature. In *Letters to a Young Doctor*, he reminds us that "the events of the body lie outside the precincts of language".

This is paradoxically a powerful argument for teaching poetry and literature – more words – to help us to look at the human condition as more than just a complex machine which may go wrong and needs some clever tinkering to put it right. In the same preface Selzer also invites us to consider "flesh as the spirit thickened".

If there is anything in this view of Selzer's, then consideration of the spirit and the tools to understand it must be important for doctors.

When doctors do become aware of these wider aspects of their work – that not all that matters to human beings in distress or illness or when they are dying, lends itself to accurate description or measurement – then to have metaphors and other ways of seeing can be very helpful. The ability to step back from narrow focus on the medical model as traditionally understood can be crucial to the practice of medicine. A specific example might show how fundamental the humanities can be when we need to work with aspects of the human condition which are of great importance to the people concerned but not always thought of as the realm of medicine. From the patient's point of view the medical model may be helpful but may fall short of addressing the significance of an illness or event to them as people.

Consider a heart attack, or myocardial infarction. Here the medical understanding is very clear: blockage of a coronary artery producing ischaemic damage to myocardium with possible arrhythmia or pump failure. The treatments are also well understood and hot angioplasty, drugs and surgery all having clearly defined and effective roles proven to work. But in reality a person has also suddenly received a wound to their very being – to their heart.

Our language is filled with examples of how we associate the heart with far more than just being a pump. Of course it can be argued that these are areas outside medicine: we fix the pump if we can and the rest is over to someone else. Yet without some such understanding of these wider effects, doctors may be much less able understand just how viscerally and personally someone is affected by their illness. As well as an increased empathy for the emotional wound the patient has received, we can be alert for the later psychological or psychiatric sequelae that may result. And we will be better placed to understand why someone does, or does not, engage with follow up treatment.

A general practitioner, perhaps in this context best referred to by our old name of family doctor, will need to bring a great deal of themselves to consultations and the management of the aftermath of such life changing illnesses. The doctor's greatest gift to a patient may be the ability to unflinchingly see them, to witness them as the human being, and not just as a collection of clinical parameters to be recorded and acted upon. When I have an acute heart attack, I certainly want a doctor who can read my ECG and clinical signs: but in the aftermath I want someone who can look me in the eye and see me, and not just 'a case'.

Patients want a certain degree of technical competence of course – certainly their lawyers would demand that – but what they really value is something else. It is the ability to see someone as wider and deeper than their illness. That itself is a good reason for a doctor to know patients for a long time, years or even decades, so that they become clearly a four-dimensional person, a human being, to whom illnesses happen on the background of their personhood. They are not defined by their illness.

Poetry is a special case. It is worth considering where, and perhaps how, poetry can offer insights and help where other forms of literature cannot. For my purposes here there are two definitions of poetry that give clues to its special place in medicine. Broyard considers that "poetry might be defined as language writing itself out of a difficult situation".

I cannot think of a better qualified person to comment on poetry than T.S. Eliot who suggested in his essay "Dante".

'Genuine poetry can communicate before it is understood.'

These two reflections point to the value of poetry to medicine, coming from different viewpoints to say something similar. Medicine is a matter of careful analysis with ceaseless striving for exactitude, and careful use of language. This of course is right and proper – indeed lifesaving. Such exactitude is vital in, for instance, discussion between specialists in an intensive care unit. There are countless examples of clarity of language being necessary in medicine, as in other specialised areas of expertise.

But to try and capture too much of the fuzziness of human feeling or experience in carefully weighed words can be futile. It may be worse than futile when our quest to compartmentalise, to capture meaning, leads us to a spurious exactitude where we believe we have defined something exactly but are in fact deceiving ourselves. This self-deception can isolate or even harm our patients. "I know how you feel" we might say because a patient has used a word or phrase that we think we understand, even a commonplace word such as 'depression'. Yet we may have wholly misjudged the interior world of the person who has been talking to us. A.A. Milne has his character Winnie the Pooh seize this problem as well as anyone when he suggests that "you find sometimes that a Thing which seemed very Thingish inside you is quite different when it gets out into the open and has other people looking at it".

Poetry can help us here, at least to understand some of the limitations of language. Indeed, it can be at its most powerful and useful just when language is failing to communicate, when the exact meaning of words, which has hitherto been so useful, suddenly has its own inadequacy cruelly exposed.

Poetry can help doctors, and others, to understand a little more of the implications behind individual medical events. Miroslav Holub, a Czech poet and immunologist, wrote a great deal of poetry that seemed to be at ease with these ambiguities and uncertainties where language and human drama intersect, at times very painfully. His poetry, it seems, lends itself well to translation into English and is the richer for the juxtaposition of medical terminology and poetry to the extent of even entitling a poetry collection *Inteferon*. One example of using poetry to make us pause when considering death and dying is this poem from that collection.

The Dead

After his third operation, his heart
riddled like an old fairground target,
he woke up on his bed
and said: Now I'll be fine,
fit as a fiddle. And have you seen horses coupling?

He died that night.

And another dragged on through eight insipid years
like a river weed in an acid stream,
as if pushing up his pallid
skewered face over the cemetery wall.

Until that face eventually vanished.

Both here and there the angel of death
quite simply stamped his hobnailed boot
on their medulla oblongata.

I know they died the same way.
But I don't believe that they are
dead the same way.

Miroslav Holub, 1968

   Does this mean that doctors need to be able to quote or
read poetry to their patients? No. There might be rare
occasions where some doctors may indeed choose do that but

I am not suggesting it here. What I am advocating is using poetry as a tool to help us, as CS Lewis suggests:

"Misunderstand a little less completely" to recognise when silence is better than words.

This has been understood clearly by Richard Selzer, who has given us the priceless gift of using words like 'love' in medicine. In *Mortal Lessons*, he does this with a clear, authoritative and wholly unsentimental tone.

'It is to search for some meaning in the ritual of surgery, which is at once murderous, painful, healing and full of love.'

These insights may help us in various ways. Rarely is there a clear answer such as one would expect in, say, an explanation of cross matching blood or reading an X-ray for instance. But always there is an equivalent of a tap on the shoulder, a gentle suggestion to consider another way of looking at things. Perhaps too there is nourishment for the spirit: doctors sorely need such nourishment.

So where does this leave the concept of dignity? This has been a constant companion on my medical journey: treating patients with dignity, trying to preserve their dignity despite the many assaults on it by illness, injury and debility. This idea of dignity is really important but narrow, reflecting as it does frequently held ideas of appearance, control of fate and functions, respect, being treated seriously as having agency. These are largely external and physical ways of assessing dignity and no one would argue against them. Yet, over time, I have been allowed to see something less easy to define but deep and enduring. If we value people for all that is human about them and recognise that they matter just because they are human, then that can be a very resilient concept. Such an attitude will transcend assaults that we might normally consider incompatible with dignity: incontinence, brain failure, delirium, or total dependence on others. It is the livening embodiment of Immanuel Kant's dictum that people are always ends in themselves.

Harvey Chochinov, a Canadian doctor, has worked to make these ideas more than just words. His 'ABCD of dignity conserving care' is about real, practical ways for doctors (and other healthcare workers) to make important differences to our patients. He writes that "how patients perceive themselves to be seen is a powerful mediator of their dignity".

It is well worth accessing the open access original paper or the British Medical Journal articles based on his work for the full details, but some examples are so helpful, so clear, that they are worth mentioning here.

'Treat contact with patients as you would any potent and important clinical intervention.'

Back to Paul Dieppe's placebo/nocebo discussion: every encounter a doctor has with a patient has the power to help them, or to harm them, even if 'nothing' is done. Or maybe especially when 'nothing' is done.

'Always ask the patient's permission to perform a physical examination.'

This is the most obvious thing but still neglected. 'Please may I listen to your chest?' Then waiting until they say, 'Yes,' before moving to do so. They always, always, say yes, and it takes literally a second or two longer but the respect it shows the patient is immeasurable. Chochinov also has much more advice, all practical and all worth noting. And it can all be incorporated into any medical practice.

Earlier I casually referred to something as being 'left brained' in rather a pejorative way. One of the most important changes to the way that I thought about the world, and medicine's place in it, has come from the work of psychiatrist Iain McGilchrist, notably his magnum opus 'The Master and His Emissary'. He has looked very carefully into the differences between the ways our left and right brains work. His book is a surprisingly easy read, despite being extremely rigorous and well referenced, and his TED talk is very watchable. Essentially, he suggests the left side of our brains (the Emissary) gives detailed attention to stuff we already know matters. It is concerned with process, measurement, decontextualised examination of fixed things. But the right side of the brain (the Master) is about much broader, sustained attention that sees things in context and makes connections, it is concerned with metaphor and wisdom. McGilchrist suggests that both medicine and the Western world have become very left brain. We are obsessed with process, detail, measurement and spurious certainty without understanding the broader contexts and the whole. The Master has given way to the Emissary.

This was a revelation to me and explained so much that I had found difficult about medicine. So often we find left brain solutions to left brain problems and this results in a demoralising strait jacket of more regulation and more process – which misses the problem completely. Once you start looking at healthcare with an eye to the different hemispheres of the brain and their different functions, then it becomes much easier to see where it has gone wrong, and why sometimes the attempts to fix it are doomed.

An extreme example of this was the revolting debacle of Mid Staffordshire Hospital. There were truly shocking things that happened there and it seems they were to a significant extent a result of a left-brain way of looking at the job of the hospital and the jobs of people who worked in it. They were not bad people, they were the same mixture of humans as found in other, excellent, places. But some of the reaction to this has been yet more left brain thinking: more regulation, more process. Courses for compassion rather than stepping back to consider why good people who went into their work for good reasons ended up lacking compassion and doing bad things. This is but one, albeit extraordinary, example of how some of the apparently extraneous things that I have bumped into over the last forty-three years in medicine really matter and can help us to make important changes for the better in healthcare.

Afterword

'Out beyond ideas of wrongdoing and right doing, there is a field. I'll meet you there.' – Rumi, *A Great Waggon*

This book was started some time ago when the world was as normal as we can ever expect it to be. It has been over 45 years in gestation, ever since I saw dimly how much power there was in kindness and how patients helped their doctors when their energy was failing. They even helped me, a slightly bewildered medical student doubting if I would ever become a doctor.

Now it is finished. I write this as I wait for the NHS to decide where to put me to help with the COVID-19 pandemic that so many doctors like me have come out of retirement to help with.

The same questions go through my mind as when I was that young student. Will I know enough, be any use, be brave enough, be kind enough? I go over my lectures I gave to medical students and junior doctors a few years ago and hope things have not changed too much.

I know one thing: It is a sick doctor that is not healed by his patients.

Bibliography

Against Empathy: The Case for Rational Compassion, Paul Bloom, Penguin Random House 2018

A Fortunate Man, John Berger and Jean Mohr. Penguin 1967, Republished Royal College General Practitioners 2003

Basic Verities, Charles Peguy, Pantheon Books Inc. 1943

Being Mortal, Atul Gawande, Profile Books, 2014

Blue Highways, William Least Heat Moon, Little Brown and Company 1982

Catharsis: On the Art of Medicine, Andrzej Szczeklik, University of Chicago Press, 2005

Death and the Afterlife, Samuel Scheffler Oxford University Press 2013

Four Quartets, TS Eliot, Faber & Faber, 2001

Genesis and Development of a Scientific Fact, Ludwik Fleck, The University of Chicago Press, 1979

Intelligent Kindness: Reforming the Culture of Healthcare, John Ballatt and Penelope Campling, RCPych Publications 2011

Intoxicated by My Illness, Anatole Broyard, Clarkson Potter 1992

Letters to a Young Doctor, Richard Selzer, Harcourt Brace & Company 1982

Living with the Devil, Stephen Batchelor, Riverhead Books 2004

Matters of Life and Death, Iona Heath, Radcliffe Publishing Ltd 2008

Moderated Love: A Theology of Professional Care, Alastair V Campbell, SPCK 1984

My Affair with Christianity, Lionel Blue, Hodder & Stoughton 1998

Poems Before & After, Miroslav Holub, Bloodaxe Books 2006

Raging with Compassion, John Swinton, Wm B Eardmans Publishing 2007

Rumi – Selected Poems, Coleman Barks, Penguin Classics 2004

Sacred Space: Right Relationship and Spirituality in Healthcare, Stephen G Wright and Jean Sayre-Adams, Sacred Space Publications 2009

Spirituality in Patient Care, Harold G Koenig, Templeton Press 2007

The Cosmic Hologram, Jude Currivan, Inner Traditions 2017

The Death of Ivan Illych & Other Stories, Leo Tolstoy, Wordsworth Classics 2004

The Human Effect in Medicine, Michael Dixon and Kieran Sweeney, Radcliffe Medical Press 2000

The Master and His Emissary, Iain McGilchrist, Yale University Press, 2009

The Solace of Fierce Landscapes, Belden C Lane, Oxford University Press 1998

The Spirituality Revolution, David Tacey, Brunner-Routledge 2004

The Structure of Scientific Revolutions, Thomas Kuhn, The University of Chicago Press, 1962